To my boys:
Brendan,
Caiden & Logan

National Library of Australia Cataloguing-in-Publication entry

Author: Westley, Renae

Title: My Vegetarian Lunchbox

ISBN: 9780994412621

Subject: Cooking, Food, Vegetarian

Dewey Number: 641.5636

Illustrations by Elena Medvedeva. Photography by Renae Westley. The publisher has done its utmost to attribute the copyright holders of all the visual material used. If you nevertheless think that a copyright has been infringed, please contact the publisher.

Published by: Of The World Publishing
ACN 133 333 141
PO Box 8070
Bendigo South LPO VIC 3550

www.oftheworldbooks.com

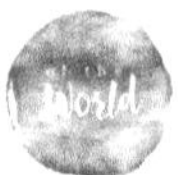

my vegetarian lunchbox

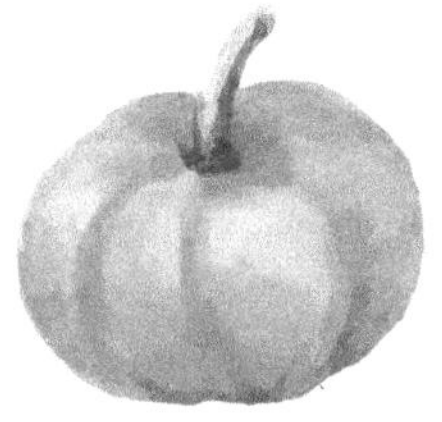

RENAE WESTLEY

Contents

6
BECOMING A VEGETARIAN
Why I chose to become a vegetarian – and how I made the change.

14
PREPARATION
Planning your meals and getting organised to make lunchtime easy.

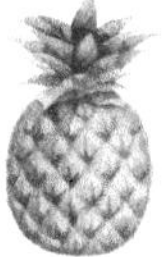

24
SUMMER
Fresh and light lunches for warmer weather.

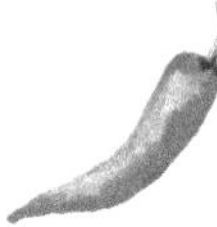

38
AUTUMN
Seasonal lunch options as the temperature starts to cool down.

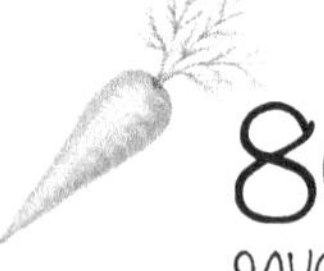

80
SAVOURY RECIPES
Fill your lunchboxes with some of my special recipes.

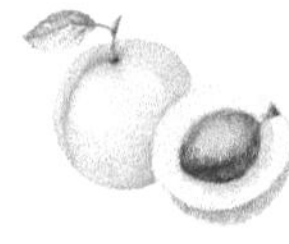

96
SWEET RECIPES
A sweet treat to finish off your meal.

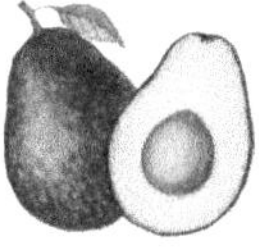

18
PANTRY BASICS
All you need to create a yummy vegetarian lunch (aside from the veggies!)

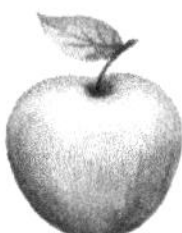

22
THE PERFECT BOX
Finding packaging to make your lunch both practical and pretty.

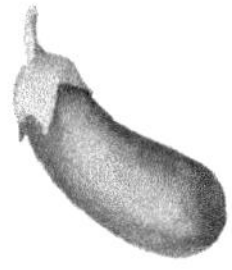

52
WINTER
Filling and comforting lunch choices for colder days.

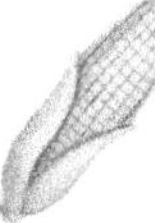

66
SPRING
Tasty, in-season treats to enjoy as the sun comes out again.

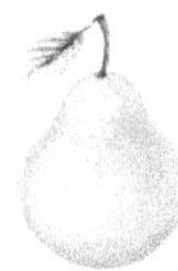

124
CONDIMENTS
Dressings & sauces to add zing to your salads.

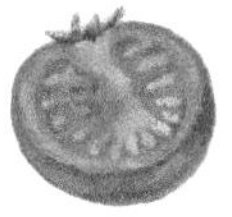

128
INDEX
Find all you need with a simple ingredients list.

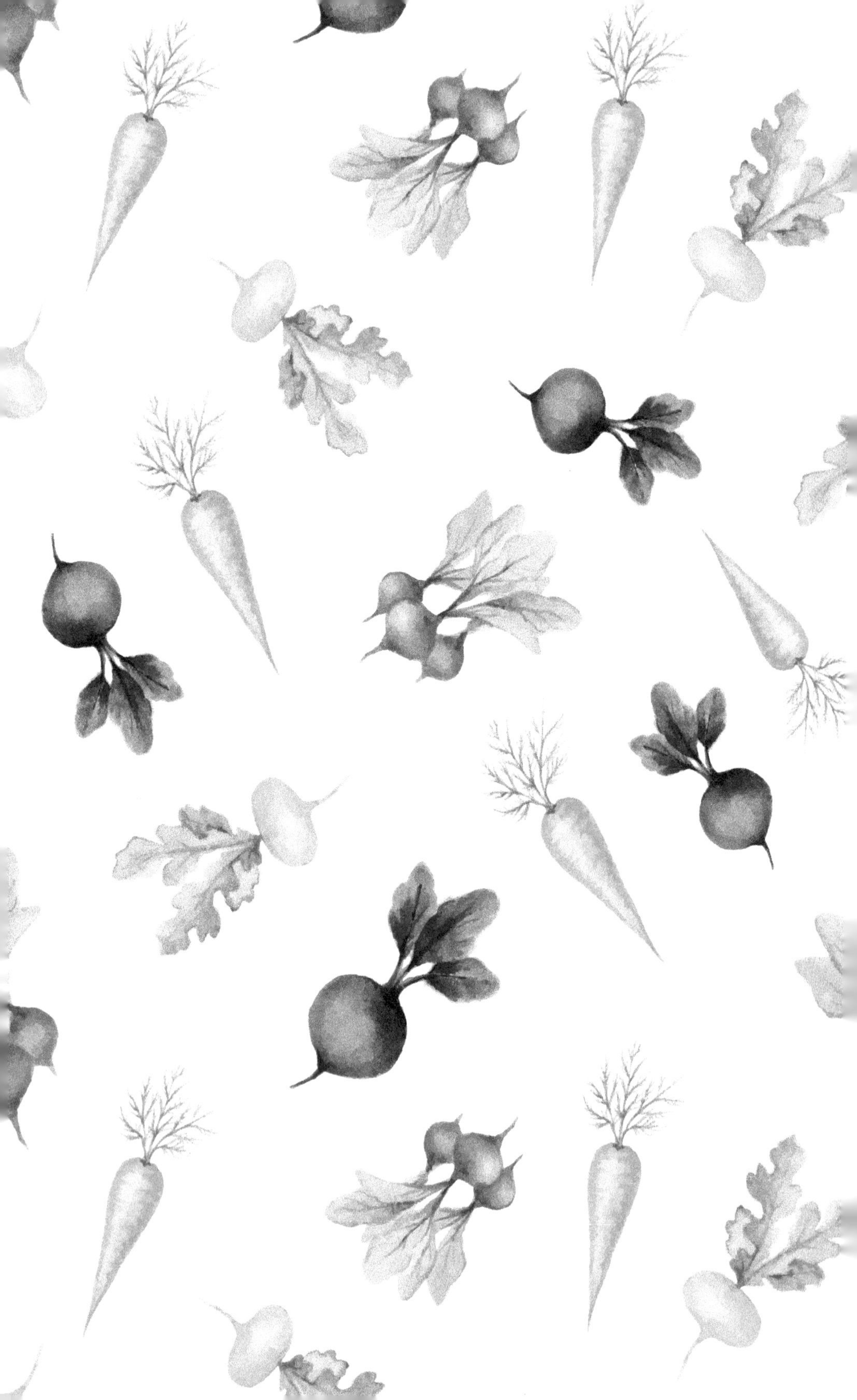

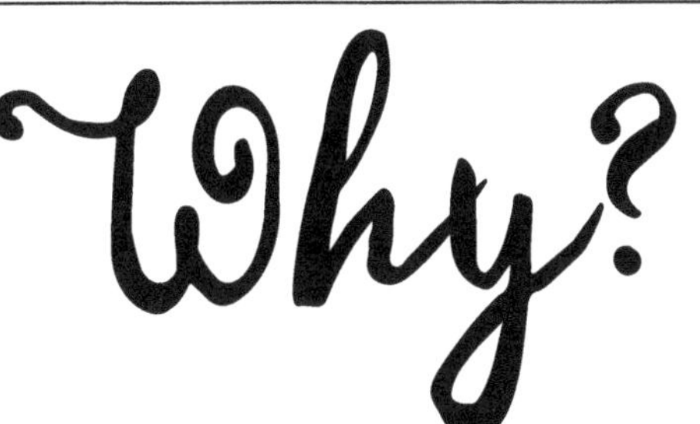

I am often asked about my path to becoming a vegetarian and how I manage daily life as a vegetarian - especially when the men in my family all enjoy the odd meat dish! Everyone's journey is very different, but this is my story.

Many people struggle with the idea of becoming a vegetarian because they are worried about how it will fit in with their lifestyle, or how they will manage the change in their diet. I promise you - it doesn't need to be a huge compromise. In the chapter ahead, I will share my journey with you and hopefully encourage you to take a few risks with food...just like I have! I hope you too will discover how beautiful and tasty vegetarian food can be.

Being a vegetarian is more exciting than just eating lettuce or spinach for three meals a day! If I can convince my husband, a big meat-eater, to enjoy a daily vegetarian lunch, then I think you will enjoy a change too!

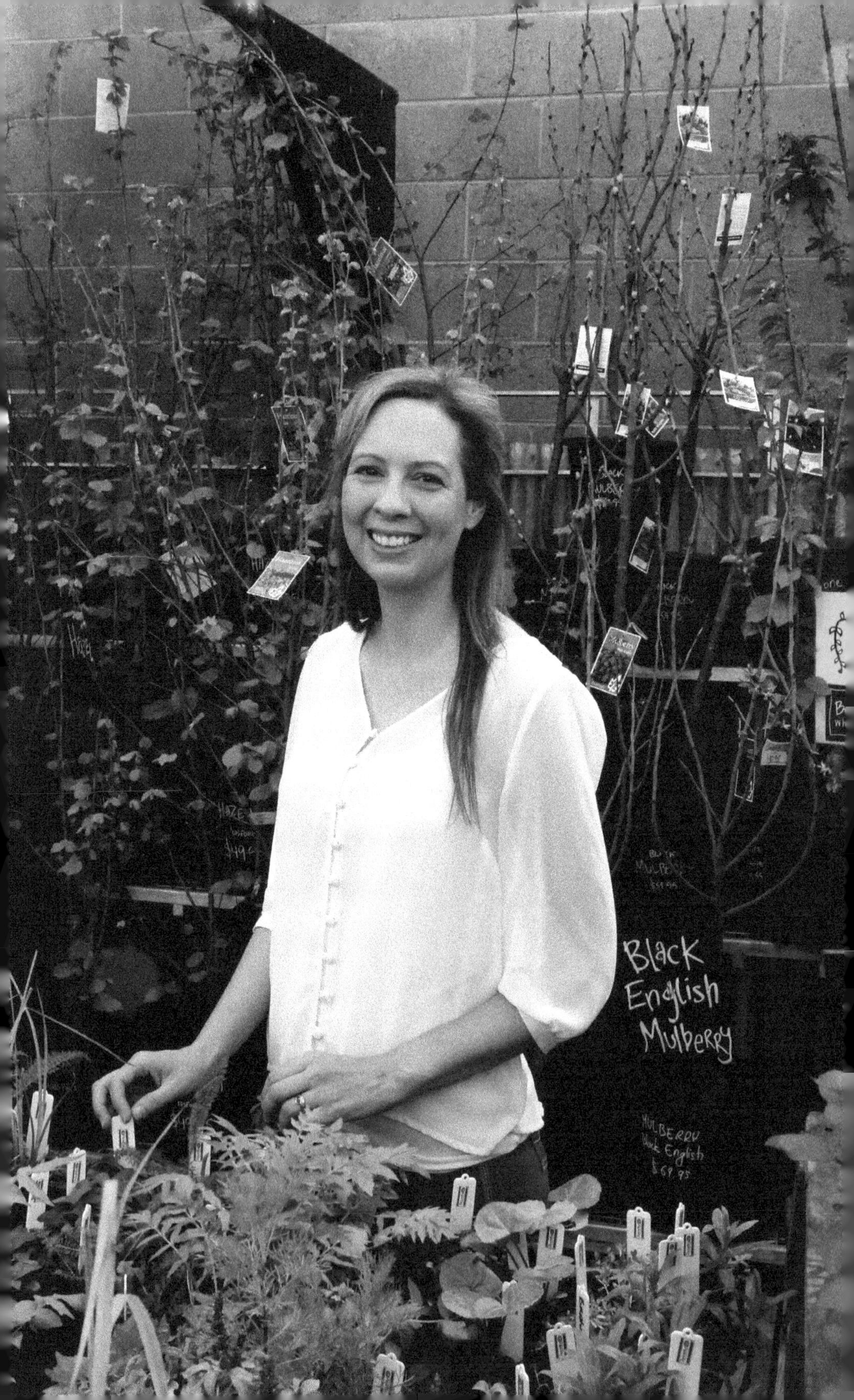
Black
English
Mulberry

Life of a vegetarian

A lot of people find it unusual when I tell them that no one else in my family is a vegetarian. Despite this, growing up I was never much of a meat-eater or a milk-drinker so it wasn't such a strange transition for me.

Growing Up

No one else in my family is a vegetarian, and I wasn't raised as one. My mother and my aunt often say that I eat like my grandmother – she wasn't a big meat-eater either. I've always been surrounded by people who appreciate and create beautiful food. My mother is an amazing cook (and Dad has just perfected the felafel!) We grew up on home-cooked meals and my brothers and I were fortunate to enjoy a balanced diet and were exposed to a variety of foods. My Nana is from the Ukraine and I remember eating khrustyky (similar to donuts), pierogi, cabbage rolls and her delicious soups. My Grandmother's baking was her specialty. I remember her making beautiful cakes and, my favourite, honey jumble biscuits. I still make those for my boys now.

My Nana and Poppy had an amazing vegetable garden. They grew vegetables and fruit and preserved them – I will never forget their massive peach tree. I remember eating freshly shelled peas from their garden too. My parents also had a small vegetable patch and freshly picked corn was a favourite. My mum was into healthy eating and home-cooking and things like white bread or soft drink were a rare treat.

I was never really a fan of meat. I gradually eliminated foods from my diet as a child – I remember eating a party pie in a lunch order at school when I was younger and finding a grisly lump. I never ate one again. I stopped drinking milk when I was about 10 as I didn't like the taste, or how it made me feel. By the time I was a teenager I only ate lean meat, or went without.

One of my closest friends became a vegetarian in high school and years later it was her who invited me away on a meditation retreat...which became the final push for me to become a vegetarian.

Stories and articles on animal cruelty have always had a strong impact on me. I remember when I was younger I would sneak down to the dams to free yabbies from the yabby nets before they could be eaten and I still want to cry now when I see animals travelling on a cattle truck. When I was younger, it was easy to disconnect between actual animals and the trays of meat in the supermarket. I didn't have to see what happened between the farm and the store. However, as my awareness grew so did my realisation that I wanted to actively do something so I started eating less meat.

The final push

When my friend, Yvonne, first asked me to attend a meditation retreat with her I was slightly bemused. I'd never meditated in my life and I had never even thought about it. A weekend away in the Dandenong Ranges with a good friend sounded lovely though, so I said yes.

It was amazing. I learnt about meditation, being self-reflective and I loved talking with the variety of people who also attended. The retreat was run by Buddhist monks so the menu was all vegetarian. I remember sending my husband a text saying 'guess what? I am eating TOFU!' but after three days I realised that I didn't miss eating meat at all.

When I got home, I decided to see how long this 'vegetarian thing' would last and, a decade later, here we are! It's been such a wonderful decision for me. The benefits have been significant and, honestly, I can't see myself ever eating meat again.

Making The Change

As I began to adapt to a vegetarian diet I found I was also making healthier choices. I became more aware of what I was eating and putting in my body. I began to read food labels and I started researching different foods, which gave me a better understanding of what we were eating.

My boys were quite young when I decided to become a vegetarian and, as the mother of young children, I had always based our family meals around kid-friendly options. My family ate (and still eat) meat, vegetables, rice and pasta however once I'd made the decision to be a vegetarian, I had to think about my meals separately from everyone else's. This was an eye-opening experience and I spent a lot of time learning to create the perfect diet for me. It made me rethink my whole approach to food and I was able to adapt my diet to suit my own appetite and my body's needs.

I'd never eaten much dairy, but I became aware that I didn't feel great when I ate it, so I cut most of it out of my diet. I also became aware of feeling heavy and bloated after eating foods like bread and pasta – so I reduced the amount of these in my diet. I started eating more whole foods, refined sugar alternatives and cleaner versions of old favourites. I lost a few kilograms quickly and around this time I also started long-distance running. Becoming a vegetarian didn't just change my diet, it changed my entire lifestyle.

Challenges

Of course, there were a few challenges in the beginning. It wasn't hard to stop eating meat – I didn't miss it at all – but making this new lifestyle work with my existing way of life was difficult. Eating meat is convenient. It was hard catering to two dietary preferences in one household for each evening meal. I had always based my meals around the meat. The vegetables were almost an afterthought. I had to rethink how I cooked and how I viewed a 'main meal'. For me, vegetables had to become the star of the show rather than the 'sides' the rest of my family were having. In the beginning, I ate a lot of the same meals my family were eating…just without the meat. This was a good starting point, but I craved more variety.

Another challenge was that my family were not prepared to come on this journey with me. My husband grew up on a farm and his views on meat are completely different to mine. He has not skipped the farm-to-supermarket step. He knows exactly where meat comes from and because of this he prefers to source and prepare a lot of the meat he and the boys eat himself. Usually, I only buy one pack of meat in our entire fortnightly shop.

The fact that we have such opposing views

puzzles many people and, yes, it can be a challenge. I find it difficult and sad when my husband brings meat home, or that I have to buy it at all when I shop, but in the end I can only make decisions for myself. However, I do need to credit my family. They too have made changes to their diet, eating far more vegetarian meals than they did in the past and they have developed their own knowledge of healthier food choices. We always find ways to make it work and if we ever go somewhere and there isn't a vegetarian option for me, I think my husband gets more upset than I do!

One of the big challenges I deal with is that my appetite doesn't compare with that of active, growing teenage boys. It can be quite difficult to find a vegetarian meal suitable for our entire family. Often, I'll make something like a vegetable curry with a big serve of rice or naan bread on the side, or perhaps a veggie stir fry with tofu for me and extra noodles for them. It helps we are all adventurous with food and the boys will always try new things. I have had some epic fails though. My first attempt at quinoa risotto was so awful we fed it to the neighbour's horse and we had toasted cheese sandwiches for dinner! The boys still joke they feel sorry for the horse.

The best way I have found to cater for everyone is through planning and organisation. We needed to develop a system and, after a bit of trial and error, we now have a great one.

Vegetarian rules?

There is definitely a perception that vegetarian and vegan lifestyles are very rigid. I classify myself as a vegetarian but sometimes labels just don't work. Some people are pescatarians (with a vegetable diet, but also eat fish and seafood). Others are vegetarian just a few days of the week (Meat-free Monday is quite popular).

There's no rule book. I make decisions every day and I try to make ethical choices I feel comfortable with. For example, I don't eat eggs - but I do use them in cooking. I make sure they're free-range, either my own or from a friend. If I buy cheese, I try to find one that is rennet-free. I don't drink milk, or eat ice cream, but I do love chocolate.

Another grey area is hidden animal products. Lollies contain gelatine. Parmesan cheese contains rennet. Worcestershire sauce contains anchovies. I am less strict here - sometimes I eat these foods, sometimes I don't.

The vegan and vegetarian community is very diverse and there will always be someone who will disagree with you. My goal is to support and inspire people who choose to enjoy vegetarian food, rather than criticise or judge someone for their choice. I congratulate anyone who has made a positive choice that is right for them.

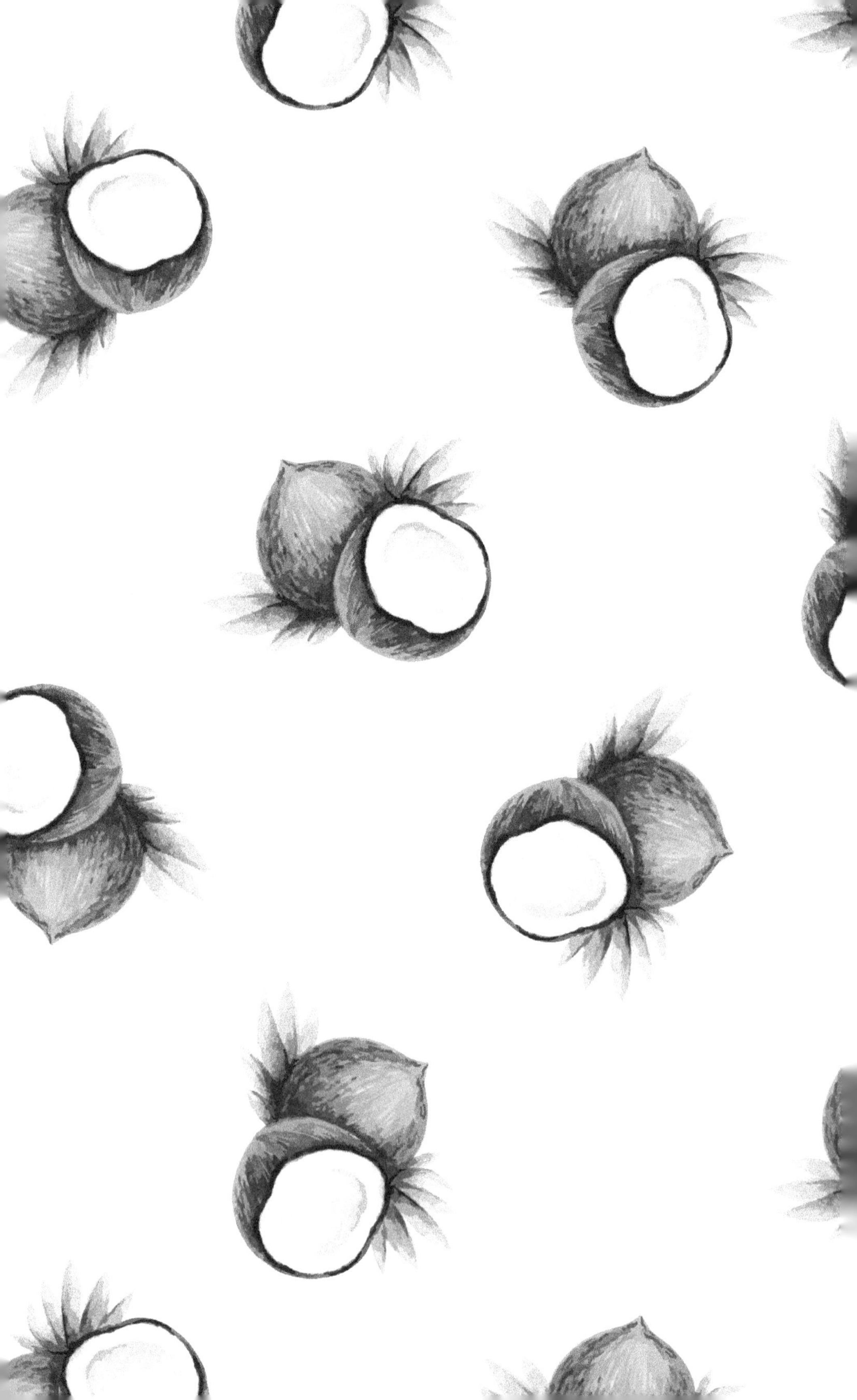

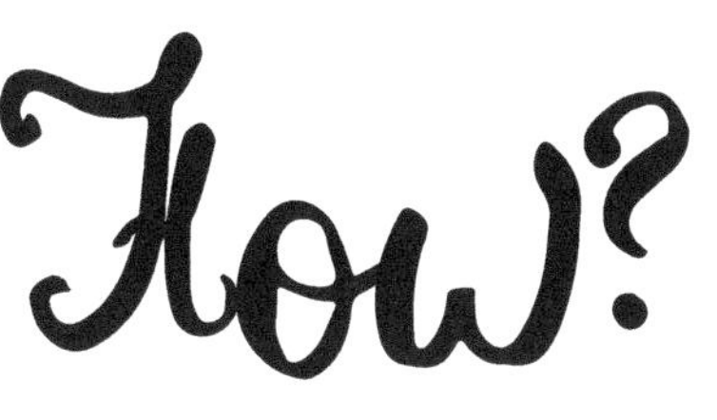

How?

I mentioned in the previous chapter that making my vegetarian life work has a lot to do with systems and planning. We lead busy lives. My husband and I both work full-time and our boys participate in a range of activities after school. Plus, we both try to find time to exercise several times a week so to try and prepare two different, nutritious meals on top of this can be quite chaotic.

I now create a fortnightly meal planner, and I have a few other tips and tricks that make life so easy when it comes to creating vegetarian meals.

Initially, my family teased me about the meal planner, but now I think they secretly love it. If I ever stray from it, they pull me up: "This wasn't on the meal planner!" Or, if they're planning on going out, they will check the planner first to see if they're missing anything!

all about the prep

When it comes to cooking for a family (who are not vegetarian) as well as creating my own yummy meals, I find that planning is the one thing that keeps life on track. I have a few little tips and tricks that make things easy and, dare I say it, even enjoyable!

Creating a meal planner

When it comes to planning, my first step is working out who in the family is at which activity each night. Now that the boys are older, we are lucky to have a couple of nights a week where all four of us sit down to eat together. When they were little, we did this every night, so these nights are quite special now.

Then I lock in at least three vegetarian meals for the fortnight. Usually this is every Wednesday and every second Sunday. Wednesday is often referred to as 'where's the meat Wednesday?' as this was the question I was asked a lot in the beginning!

Something I find helpful is planning to cook extra serves of meat-based meals. I designate the number of servings on the meal planner so that I have enough for a 'left overs' night. On those nights, I get to really focus on a vegetarian meal for me. I also try to use the slow cooker at least once a fortnight and that also allows me to just focus on my meal at the end of the day.

Finally, once a fortnight we also have a 'fend for yourself night' where I don't worry about anyone except myself. We all cook and eat whatever we feel like and it's often something quick and easy – like baked beans on toast! I often make this night on a Friday and that means I have more time to sit down and do something else...like creating my meal planner for the coming fortnight!

Off to the shops

Once I've planned the fortnight, I check what ingredients I need in order to make the meals and see what's in the cupboard so I can make a shopping list. The following Saturday morning I will go to a large supermarket to get mostly non-perishable items. Once I've completed the supermarket shop, I head to the whole foods store and pick up all my specialty products – coconut yoghurt, cheeses, dips, kombucca, anything else that perhaps catches my eye.

The local Farmers' Market is held on the second Saturday of every month where I live (one day I hope it will be more often!) and that usually coincides with one of my fortnightly shops. From there, I will try to buy as many seasonal fruits and vegetables as I can. I often don't plan my vegetarian meals. It's exciting to find fresh produce and create meals around them. Each Sunday there is another local market and my husband and I enjoy going there to get produce as well.

Through the week, I try not to go to the supermarket unless I absolutely have to. If we are out of bread, milk, pet food or apples, I will go. It all sounds great in theory, but I still feel like I am at the supermarket a lot!

Some weeks are better than others.

Lunch preparation

When it comes to lunch preparation, I try and complete some of that ahead of time. I usually have a raw slice (see page 118), bliss balls (see page 116) or a 'cheesecake' (see page 110) in my freezer. This allows me to have snacks on hand and ready to pop into a lunchbox. I take it out of the freezer the night before and store it in the fridge overnight ready to pack in the lunchbox in the morning with minimal effort. By the time the snack is ready to eat, it has thawed.

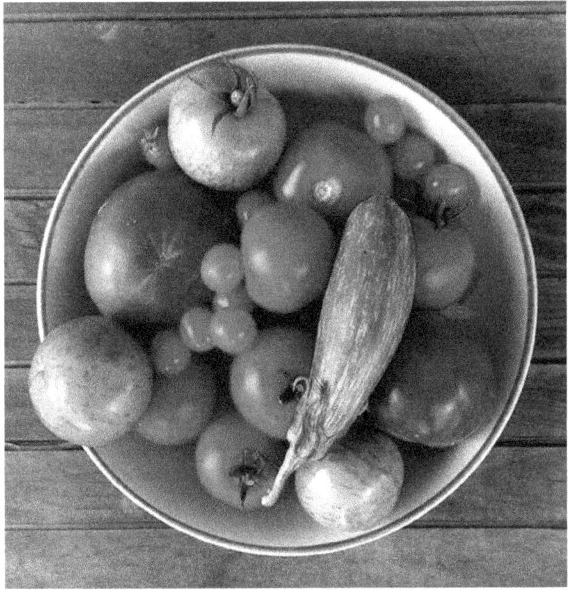

Sunday is my big day of lunchbox preparation. I put my iPod on shuffle, crank up the volume and commit to a couple of hours in the kitchen. What I will bake on a Sunday is also included on the meal planner so I know ahead of time what I am going to make and I can ensure I have the appropriate ingredients on hand.

On Sunday I usually make two items for lunches that week. One is super healthy and the other a little more indulgent (as you will find in the 'sweet' section of this book!) If I have any large pieces of fruit – like pineapple or watermelon – I cut them into small pieces and pop them into containers, ready for lunchboxes.

I will often roast a tray of vegetables on a Sunday. These can be used in my vegetarian meals through the week, or added to salads in my lunchboxes. In winter, I will often make a pot of soup each week. Finally, I make our salads for the next day's lunch. I used to put the salad dressing on in the morning, but now I find it is best to put them in their own container so they can be tipped over just before the salad is eaten.

During the week, I think about each day's lunch when I am making dinner. Typically, I lift everything that I will be using for dinner, or that could go in a lunchbox out of the fridge and on to the bench. I then put our family dinner and lunch salads together at the same time, putting items back in the fridge as I am finished with them.

When making salads, I look to see if I can use any of the dinner ingredients – like pasta or rice – and put those in too. If we are having something like broccoli, I may steam a little extra to add to a salad.

I am often asked how I come up with salad combinations and honestly it is totally dependent on this process. Whatever I have in the veggie drawer that can go in a salad

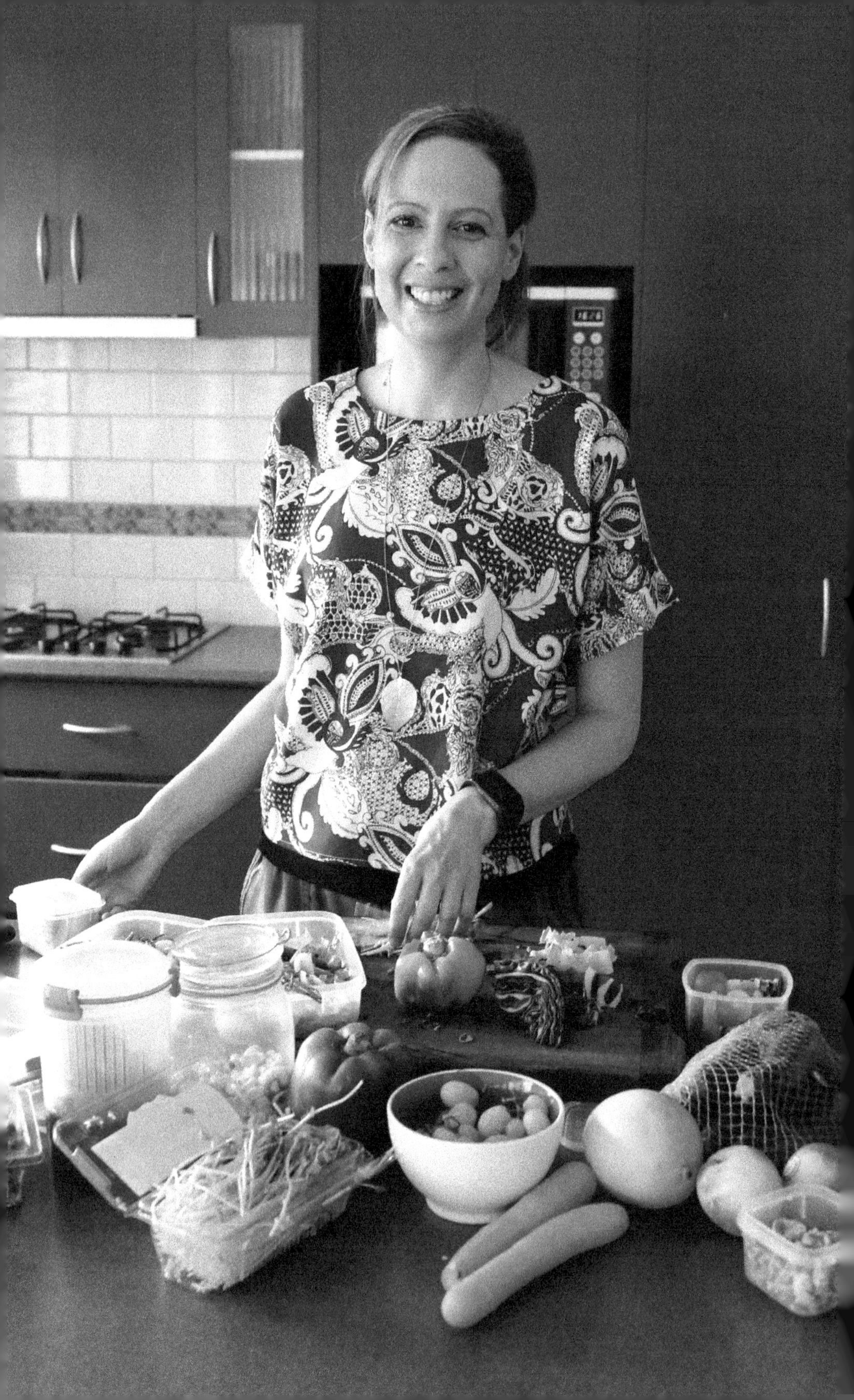

tends to go in! If the salad is looking a little sparse, I might go the pantry and use a tin of lentils or beans. Sometimes I will use vegetables from the freezer if I think I need to bulk out the salad a little more. I also keep jars of olives, artichokes and marinated capsicum handy as these always make a great addition.

In the cooler weather, I like to include some heartier foods, or foods that can be heated.

I have all our snacks set out the night before. As you will see, I like to put things in their own little containers, so chips, nuts or fruit will all go out on the bench. Everyone has their own 'spot' to help with organisation in the morning.

> I dont pack a lunch with a plan or a system in mind – it really comes together as I am doing it so I encourage everyone to experiment!

I don't pack a lunch with a plan or a system in mind - it really comes together as I am doing it, so I encourage everyone to experiment. I tend to start with a large salad or veggie combination and then add fruit, a savoury snack and a sweet snack based on what is available following all that planning. There is more information about the packing process and how I prepare the lunchboxes on page 22.

Thankfully, after all of that preparation, there is little to do in the morning. I take any items from the fridge that we need and lay them on the bench in the designated spot. If I need to make sandwiches, I do that in the morning too.

a little extra thought...

The majority of time, I find the fruit and vegetables I buy are seasonal – especially when I've shopped at the Farmers' Market. However, we live in a world where we can buy fruit and vegetables that have been grown hydroponically or which have been shipped from elsewhere, even overseas. I always look to see if fruit and vegetables are grown in Australia. I also do this with my canned produce. There are times when I will buy out of season, but my preference is locally grown, seasonal produce. The closer it is grown to my home, the better.

People often ask how I manage to eat so much when they look at my lunchboxes, but it's actually my husband's lunchbox I photograph. He has more of a selection, so it's a little more interesting to look at! Mine is a modified version of his - usually the same salad but only two snacks. As a teacher, my times to eat (like my children's) are based on what time the bell rings for recess, lunch and the end of the day. My husband is different though - he can be driving around or sitting behind a computer, so he doesn't have an eating pattern and he often craves snacks. So, I pack plenty but I try to keep them as healthy as possible. My theory is that then it doesn't matter what he chooses to eat (or how much he may eat) he will still be making a good choice and less likely to stop and snack on unhealthy options.

Pantry Basics

Part of making a vegetarian life simple is having all the things you need at your fingertips. If you have a well-stocked pantry, then you are more likely to make good choices when it comes to eating and meals.

The Staples

These are main items you will always find in my pantry. With these I can create the majority of the baking recipes in this book. This list of pantry ingredients is something I've built up over time. I buy one or two of these items each time I shop, as I need them or as they run out:

- Coconut Oil
- Desiccated Coconut
- Tahini
- Almond Meal
- Nuts
- Flours
- Baking Powder / Bi-carb Soda
- Honey
- Peanut Butter
- Sugar Alternatives
- Cacao
- LSA
- Seeds
- Puffed Rice
- Puffed Millet
- Buckinis
- Rolled Oats
- Vanilla Paste
- Dried Fruit and Berries

I always have several different kinds of nuts and they double as snacks or salad ingredients.

I also have an assortment of flours: Spelt, Brown Rice, Regular, Coconut, Besan. Different recipes call for different flours and I like to experiment with them when I cook. It is important to also have Baking Powder and Baking Soda on hand as not all flours will have a raising agent.

I have a range of sugar alternatives including rice malt syrup, agave, maple syrup, coconut syrup and coconut sugar. Many of these are interchangeable in recipes, although each has its own flavour. Of course I often use honey in place of sugar too.

There are usually several different varieties of seeds and dried fruits in my pantry. I store the seeds in small jars or add left overs to my activated seed mix.

If I have any packets with only a small amount of seeds, or some of these other ingredients, I'll tip them all into one big jar. I soak a teaspoon of this mix in water before I go to bed each night to 'activate' the seeds and nuts. I then add this to my muesli in the morning.

I don't have a standard shopping list. Our shopping list is always on the fridge so the family can add to it as things run out. I record the bulk of the things I need to buy when I create the meal planner and I usually just buy a stack of fruit and vegetables and work whatever is seasonal or available into our meals.

However, there are things I do buy almost every each week.

These include: muesli, tinned tomatoes, tinned corn, tinned legumes, dry pasta, vegetable stock, vegetable chips, basmati rice, instant brown rice, almond milk, cashews, yogurt, coconut yogurt, haloumi cheese, feta cheese and cheddar cheese.

My meals are mainly based on vegetables and fresh produce – but there are times when there are a few other things I use that I would recommend having on hand. These include:

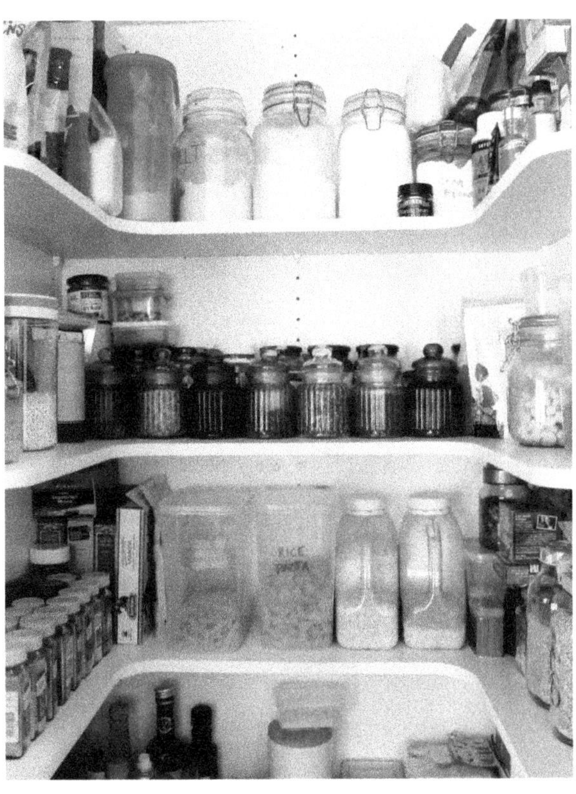

Massal Stock – this is my favourite vegetarian stock. It doesn't matter what vegetables you have, you can always turn them into a soup using this stock. I love barley in soups as well and always have this in my pantry.

Haloumi Cheese – a few slices of grilled haloumi either with salad in summer or with vegetables in winter is another quick and easy vegetarian meal.

Wraps – I often turn these into pizza bases (as I don't like the thick doughy ones) or to create salad wraps or soft tacos. Wraps can also be used to make veggie quesadillas in the sandwich press.

Miso Paste – I use this as flavouring in a range of recipes. A quick and easy meal is to put some vegetables and tofu in a bowl, add miso paste then pour over boiling water. However, miso paste does contain bonito which is a fish flavour, so it is not 100% vegetarian or vegan friendly.

Canned 4 bean mix – I find this a protein rich base I can quickly turn into a meal. It may be a salad, or the filling of a burrito or a quesadilla.

Tofu or Tempeh – I always have a pack of each in the fridge or freezer. This makes it easy to throw together a quick vegetarian stir fry, curry, salad or soup.

Instant rice – rice is my favourite grain to have for dinner. If the rest of the family is having it with their meal, it usually becomes the base of mine too. However, if they are not, I have an instant brown rice that can be heated and eaten with salad, vegetables or tofu to create a quick and filling meal.

Lentils – both canned and dry. I often used canned lentils, rinsed and drained in salads. But lentils are also great when making vegetarian versions of recipes like lasagne, Shepard's pie and Bolognese.

Fritters – all you need on hand to make fritters is flour and an egg or two. My whole family enjoy fritters and they are a great way to use up any veggies you have lurking in your crisper drawer.

TVP – TVP, or Textured Vegetable Protein is a soy product you can use as a meat replacement. I don't cook with it often, but I like to have it on hand, especially if I'm in the mood for vegetarian Spaghetti Bolognese.

Frozen Gyoza – I like to have a packet of vegetarian gyoza in the freezer. They only take 8 minutes to steam and are a super quick meal if I'm really caught out.

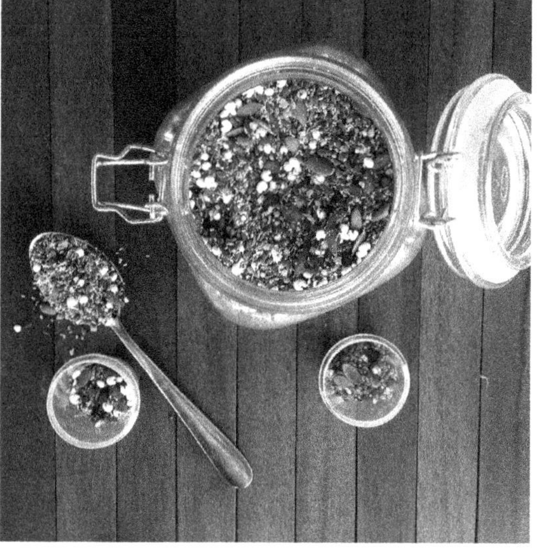

Soba Noodles – these cook quickly and can bulk out a salad to turn it into a filling meal. They are also great to add to a soup or broth in order to make it more filling.

Flavoured Salt – I love having a tray of roast veggies prepped. All I do is drizzle the vegetables with olive oil and sprinkle them with my favourite quality flavoured salt. Some of my favourites are wild herb or lemon myrtle.

Balsamic Vinegar – this is my ultimate salad dressing ingredient (as you will soon see!) I always have a bottle of both red and white balsamic in the pantry.

Sauces and Spices – I have a range of these in the cupboard and they last awhile.

Storage

I store my vegetables in the crisper drawer of the fridge. I keep fruit such as apples, pears, citrus and bananas in a fruit bowl in my kitchen (I find having them visible means the boys will often grab something on the way past which makes for a quick and healthy choice for snacking) and I store more delicate fruit such as berries and stone fruit in the refrigerator.

We go through a lot of vegetables. I usually adapt our meals each night to utilise what is in the veggie drawer. When the weekend comes, I'll look for a way to use up anything left. I might make a pot of soup that I can pack in our lunches, freeze or eat as a vegetarian meal. I may also roast a tray of vegetables I want to use up. I use these in my own vegetarian meals or in our lunch salads.

In the end, we have very little waste that is food scraps. All of our left overs are usually turned into lunches or eaten on our regular left over nights. Any scraps go to the chickens, the compost or to our dog. I always feel a sense of satisfaction when I able to use something up either in a lunch box or as a meal rather than throw it in the bin. I do not like to waste food, so I will look for ways to use things up before throwing them away.

The Backyard Supermarket

We were lucky when we moved into our current house there were established fruit trees. We have four citrus trees; two orange trees, a lemon and a lime. We also have three stone fruit trees; an apricot, peach and plum. There is also an amazing passionfruit vine that grows over our fence. We had an enormous vine at our old house and were used to a constant supply of passionfruit. These days, if you ever see a passionfruit in one of my lunch boxes, there's a chance it's come from my neighbours vine, but they drop all over the ground on our side of the fence, so I don't think they mind sharing.

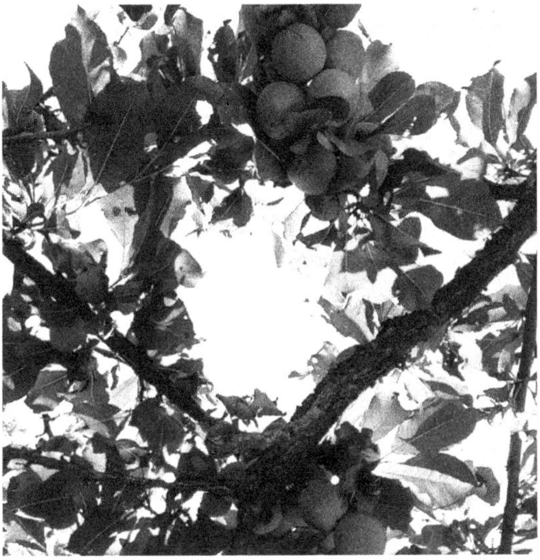

My mother is a gardener. She always has been and she is very good at it. I, on the other hand, am not a natural gardener. Up until recently any pot plant I owned had a limited life span. However, I have been working on this over the last few years. I love the idea of growing my own food and I really enjoy doing it. My mum has helped me set up a potted herb garden and with her assistance I've successfully grown a range of herbs including parsley, dill, thyme, mint, Vietnamese mint, chocolate mint, marjoram, oregano, basil, lemongrass, coriander and sage. They haven't all made it. I've had a few casualties along the way and my mother always comes over and patiently helps me to repot and replant, and I try again.

I've also grown a range of other produce in larger pots including kale, chard, lettuce, spinach, strawberries, eggplant and chillies. My biggest success has been with our tomato plants. We put in five or six during the month of November and enjoy an abundance of tomatoes for months and months.

Again, I have to credit my mother. If she didn't come and help me, my garden wouldn't be anywhere near as productive. I don't need to buy herbs or tomatoes in summer and it's lovely to supplement our grocery supplies with home-grown produce. It's also very convenient to have all of those herbs handy.

We also have a chook pen and keep up to four chooks at a time. This gives us three to four eggs a day and the chooks eat all of our food scraps, which is a win-win if you ask me.

My father-in-law keeps his own bees, so he provides us with honey from his hives. There is a hive in one of the trees in our backyard, we have tried to coax the bees into a proper hive so that we can collect honey – but the bees are happy where they are and haven't moved.

Lunchbox tips

I get asked a lot of questions about my lunchboxes so, I thought I would answer a few of them here!

Where do you find your lunchboxes?

Everywhere! This is another one of my obsessions – I have two drawers full of containers of all shapes and sizes. My most frequently asked question on Instagram is- "Where did you get your containers?" and I always feel bad that I cannot give people a brand or store where they are from.

The large container is available at many variety stores in Australia, like The Reject Shop or Big W. It is meant for slices. The salad container is from the brand **décor** and I just buy those at the supermarket – but it is widely available in Australia. One day I discovered that they fit together perfectly … and I haven't looked back.

The small containers? Well they really are from everywhere. If I am in a supermarket or variety store I can't help but look. When the 'Back to School' stock is in shops at the beginning of the school year – I'm there. Buying every shape and colour I can find. The way they fit together comes about almost by accident - it is always based on what I pack that day.

Everything fits so neatly – how can I do this?

I honestly do this by trial and error. Sometimes I look back over my own posts and think, wow that combination worked well I should try and revisit that … but I can never remember what that combination was, and as I have different snacks, it would be different anyway.

The process I usually follow is to put the salad in first. Then the sweet treat for the week. Depending on what that is or how I cut it will determine the size of that container. Next are the fruit and / or veggie sticks. Again this is dependent on what I have on hand. Once these are all in I find containers to fit the gaps. I am usually then left with two to four containers to fill. I begin looking through my savoury and other snack options. Nuts, dips, chips, dark chocolate, maybe a second serve of fruit, popcorn, dried fruit, seeds. I'll play around with ingredients until I am happy with the balance both nutritionally and visually.

Once you have put lids on all the smaller containers, does the big lid then fit?

When I first started packing these lunches, I barely used any smaller containers. I'd pack the snacks, put the lid on the container, everything would roll around everywhere and get muddled up. It was a flawed system. So I started using the smaller containers. However, I suddenly hit another road block – the lid wouldn't always fit on. Some of the containers were too high or others not high enough and the ingredients would escape again.

So, a system slowly evolved.

Once I've photographed the lunch, I put all of the small lids on the containers. I put any containers that do not need to be refrigerated on the bench. I leave everything else where it is and just sit the large container in the fridge, like a tray with the smaller ones sitting inside. In the morning, Hubby takes the big container out of the fridge and packs all of his snacks from the bench back into it. He doesn't need to put the big lid on – all the little lids are on, everything is sitting snuggly in the tray and can be carried out together then put straight into the fridge at his work. Or, if it is a hot day or he is on the road, he will take ALL of the little containers out of the tray and pack them into a cooler bag.

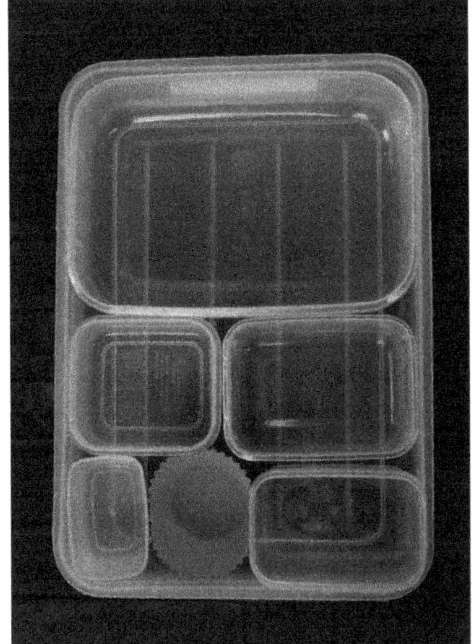

So the lunch box photos are a little bit of an illusion – I don't use a big lid at all. But the little lids do exactly the same thing and packing this way helps me to pack a consistent amount of snacks each day. Plus I like the way the final packed lunches look. I do have a taller version of the tray lunch box that I could use, but it is so high, I have the same problem I had in the beginning and have to put all the little lids on anyway – so I stick to the system I have.

Have you had any disasters on the move with your lunchbox?

Not that I can think of. My disaster stories are usually related to the new and out there foods I try and make my family eat. I once packed hubby raw broccoli soup. I'd eaten it the night before and enjoyed it but he told me it was an "epic fail." My kids often identify snacks as "healthy" – some they like, but some they won't touch.

How do you store the lunchboxes when not in use?

I have not one, but two massive drawers full of containers – and even then they don't all fit. The really large ones or ones I use to keep cakes in need to be stored elsewhere. No one in the family will attempt to put the washed containers away – they just leave them on the draining rack for me. This is probably best for all of us...

Do you have any other tips regarding storage or care of your lunchboxes?

When it comes to washing up, I am a convenience kind of person – if I can't put it in the dishwasher, it is too much effort.

However, I would advise always storing containers with their lids on. Many people I talk to say they can never find the lids when they need them. Once upon a time I was that person too. Now I don't put the container away until it has its lid. I do stack the same type of containers inside each other with all the matching lids on top. This maximises space in the drawer and makes it easier to find what I'm looking for.

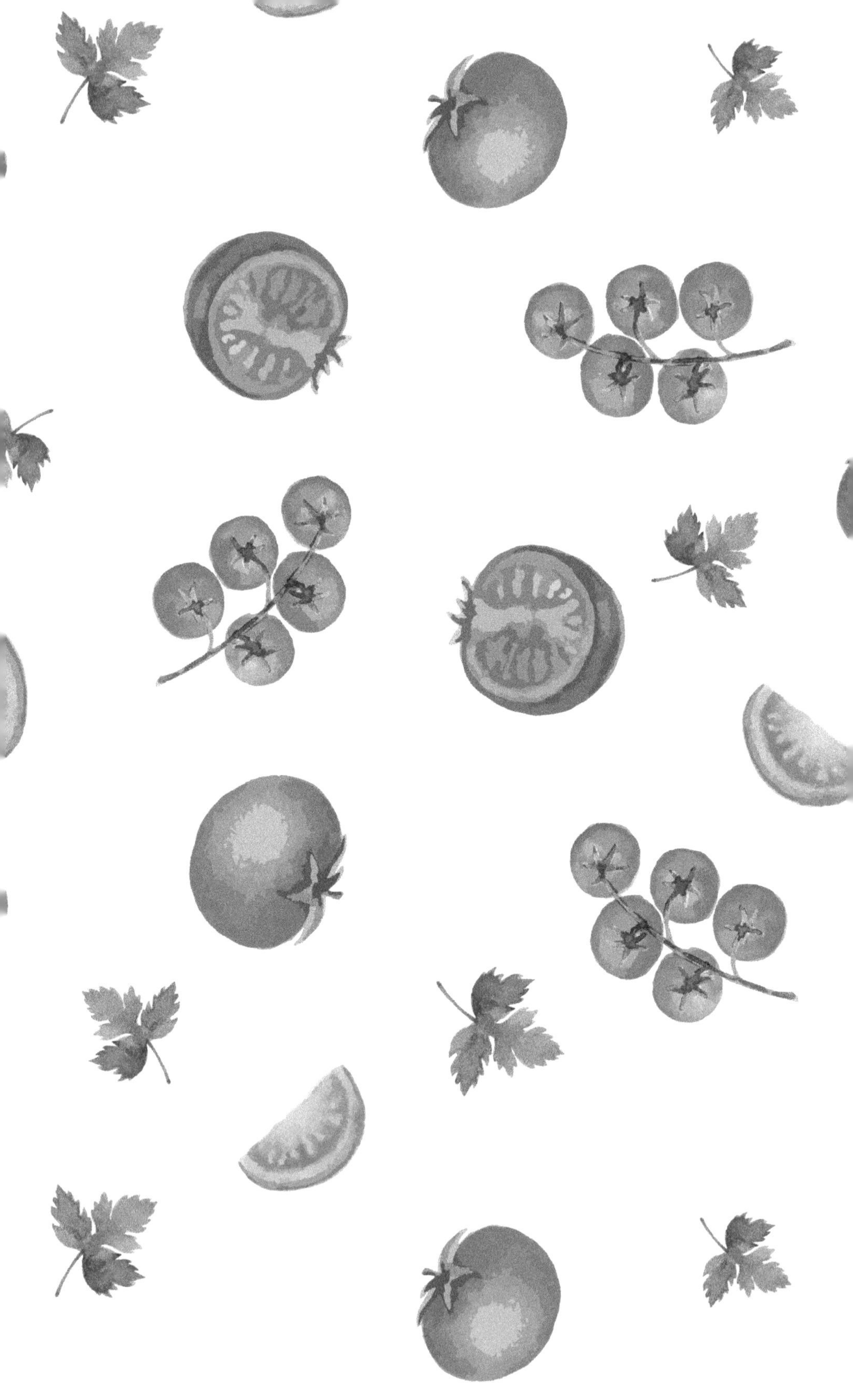

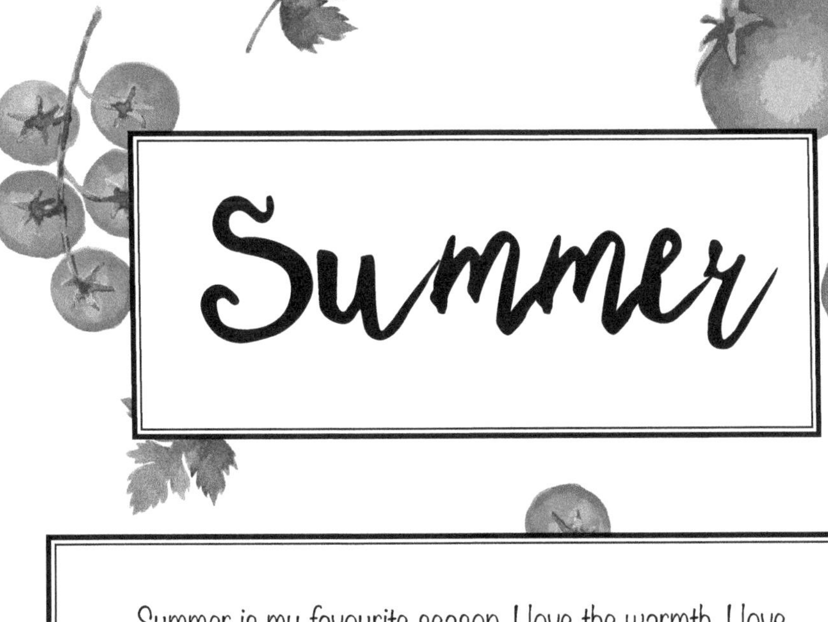

Summer

Summer is my favourite season. I love the warmth, I love being outside, and I love all those long days with extra daylight. There is something so lovely about being completely warm - not needing socks, a heat pack or the heater totally cranked up. It is rare that I complain about the heat, I soak it up like a lizard!

For me, Summer is all about eating light. It's the perfect weather for fruit and salads and I tend to make more smoothies this time of the year too. Usually, I don't like food that is really cold unless it's very hot outside. I adore stone fruit (as you will see) and it's in abundance during this time of the year so I often pack additional servings. I do miss soup in the Summer though. It's such a quick, easy and nutritious meal but it always feels a little strange to eat soup on hot days.

As well as yummy stone fruit, Summer is also the best time of the year to enjoy berries - blackberries, blueberries, raspberries and strawberries as well as melons, oranges and cherries. For cheap and abundant veggies, look out for celery, chillies, lettuce and capsicum.

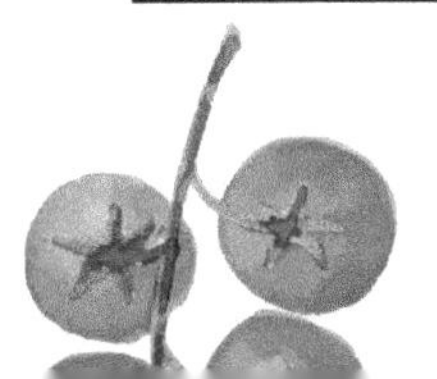

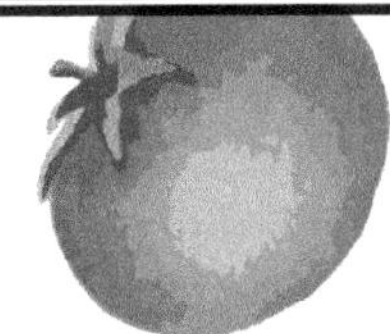

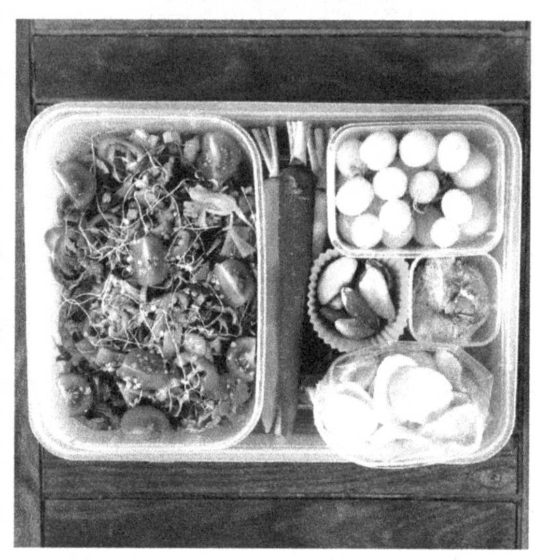

Keeping it fresh

I've always loved the idea of growing my own herbs, fruit and vegetables - but sadly I've never been a natural green thumb. Luckily my mum and my husband are willing to offer their assistance and with a little (ok, a lot) of help I've been growing a range of my own produce - including the lettuce in this salad. It is such a wonderful feeling to bring food straight from the garden in to your kitchen.

- Home grown lettuce, spinach, salad herbs, alfalfa, snow peas, red capsicum, tomato and hemp seeds, dressed with white balsamic vinegar
- Grapes
- Heriloom carrots & Pumpkin and basil dip
- Brazil nuts & Vegetable chips

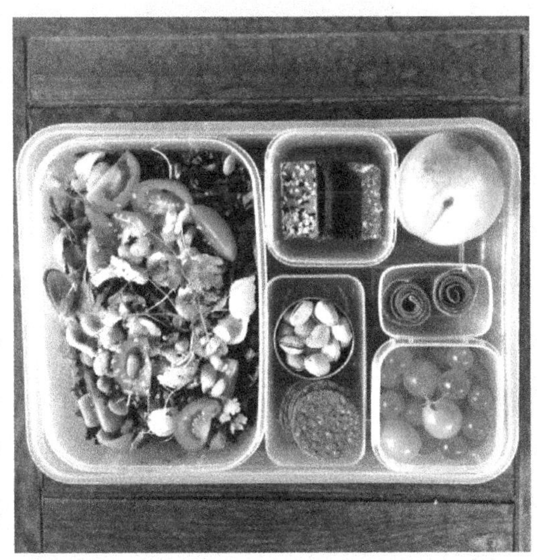

a cherry on top

Cherry tomato plants are my favourite variety to plant and grow. Once the tomatoes begin to ripen, there are new ones ready to pick almost every day. I have never tired of walking out into the garden to pick them. I almost feel like I am on an Easter Egg hunt, lifting up leaves and looking for those bright bursts of colour, even eating one or two. This lunch box celebrates them as a snack in their own right, rather than a salad ingredient.

- Salad of spinach, kale, grated beetroot, micro herbs, orecchiette pasta, tomato, edamame beans and hemp seeds, dressed with balsamic vinegar
- Black tahini slice (see page 118 for recipe)
- Fruit leather (see page 96 for recipe)
- Cherry tomatoes & Peach
- Pistachios & Black rice biscuits

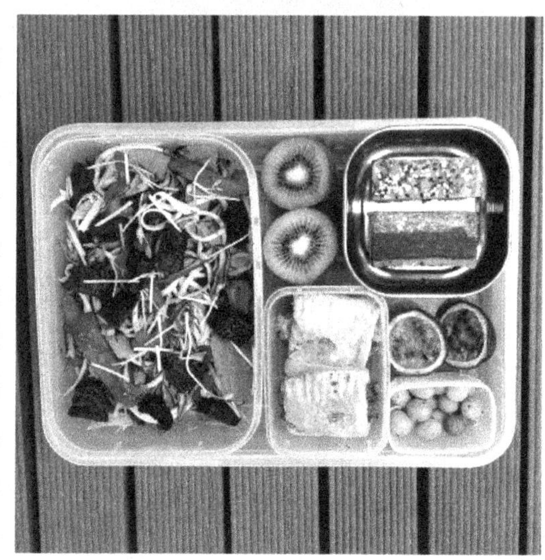

Endless possibilities

I love the endless possibilities when it comes to salads. There are so many beautiful plant-based ingredients and never ending ways to mix and combine them. I'll use leafy greens or vegetables that are raw, cooked, preserved, canned or frozen. I love adding legumes, nuts or seeds for an extra crunch. Even fruit makes a beautiful addition to a summer salad. Sometimes you just have to think outside the (lunch) box when selecting ingredients to keep your salads varied and interesting.

- Salad of lettuce, red cabbage, zucchini zoodles, roast capsicum, roasted beetroot and snow pea sprouts, dressed with white balsamic vinegar
- Veggie 'sausage' rolls (see page 82 for recipe)
- Black tahini slice (see page 118 for recipe)
- Kiwi fruit & Passionfruit
- Kri Kri (covered peanuts)

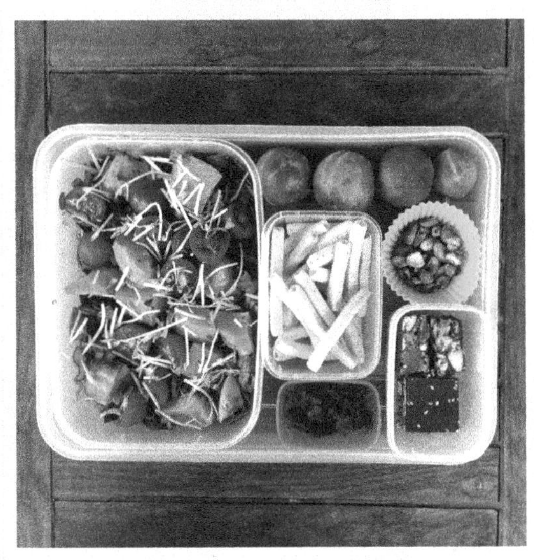

Plum good

Blood plums are a favourite fruit in our family. Years ago, my husband and I planted several fruit trees, including a blood plum, in our backyard. We nurtured them through the drought and enjoyed several seasons of beautiful fruit and plums - then, we sold the house and I was so sad to say goodbye to those trees. Luckily, the new house we bought also had several fruit trees, including a blood plum tree! It is a Summer highlight when those plums are ripe. They are just perfect in lunchboxes.

- Salad of spinach, red cabbage, red onion, roasted sweet potato, tomato and snow pea sprouts, dressed with red balsamic vinegar

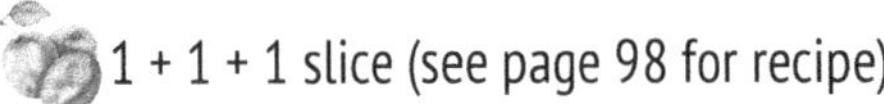

- 1 + 1 + 1 slice (see page 98 for recipe)
- Beetroot relish (see page 126 for recipe)
- Blood plums
- Pistachios & Veggie straws

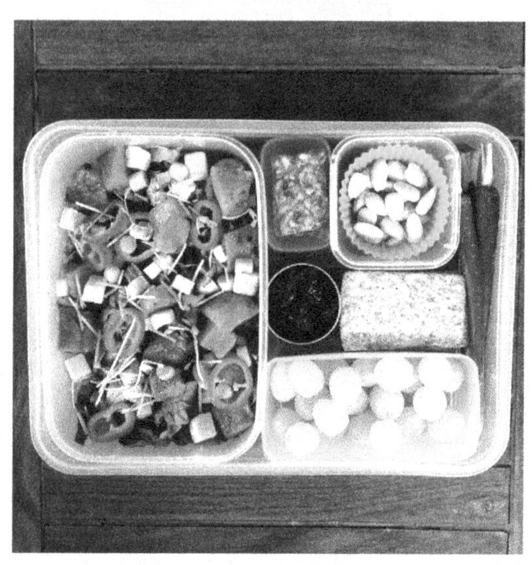

The secret ingredient

I'm going to tell you a secret. Up until recently, I didn't like pumpkin. My mum tells me that even as a baby, I would eat every pureed vegetable – except pumpkin. But my tastebuds have definitely evolved as a vegetarian (thankfully, because pumpkin is common in vegetarian recipes!) and I am always willing to try new things. On a night during a roast dinner, I bravely put a piece of pumpkin on my plate ... and, loved it! I now think that roasted pumpkin is beautiful, so much so it is a popular addition to many of my salads.

- Salad of home grown lettuce, spinach, cucumber, spring onion, tasty cheese, capsicum, roasted capsicum and snow pea sprouts, dressed with white balsamic vinegar
- Bek's date and nut slice (see page 100 for recipe)
- Beetroot relish (see page 126 for recipe)
- Grapes & Purple heirloom carrots
- Multi-grain crackers & Blanched almonds

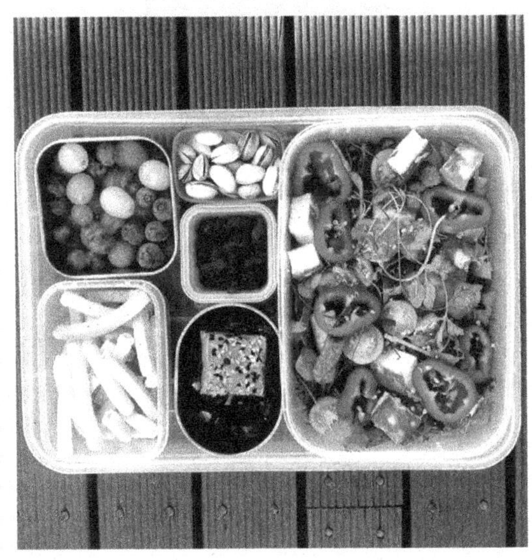

Relish the season

You may have already noticed I regularly include a little pot of beetroot relish in my lunches. This is my mum's homemade relish and it is absolutely beautiful. We always have a bottle of her homemade sauce and a jar of this relish in our fridge. Beetroot is a wonderful vegetable - it is full of vitamins and minerals, is low in fat and is packed with antioxidants.

- Salad of spinach, cabbage, micro herbs, haloumi cheese, capsicum, hemp seeds and home grown tomatoes, dressed with white balsamic vinegar
- Black tahini slice (see page 118 for recipe)
- Grapes & Blueberries
- Pistachios & Chocolate covered sultanas
- Veggie straws & Beetroot relish (see page 126 for recipe)

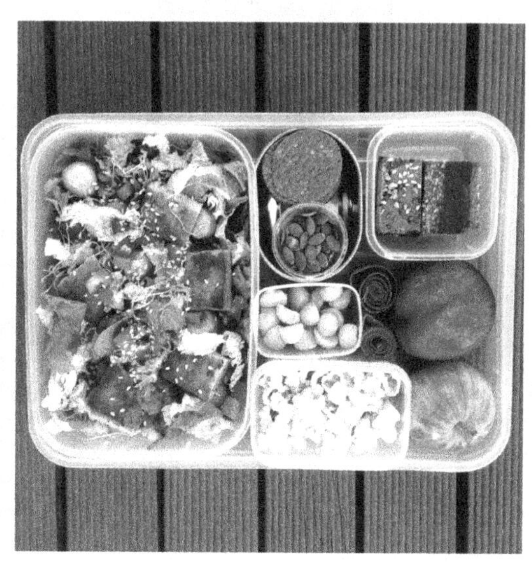

Let's talk tofu

Let's take a minute to talk about tofu. Before I was vegetarian, I avoided it like the plague. It was weird and unknown and I wanted nothing to do with it. However, being vegetarian has made me more experimental when it comes to food and cooking. When you cut out the food you used to base all of your meals around, then you need to at least try all possible replacements. So now? I really enjoy tofu! I have some good recipes up my sleeve (salt and pepper tofu, scrambled tofu, tofu stir fry...) and when I have left overs, it is great in salads!

Salad of lettuce, rice, Chinese cabbage, spring onion, tomato, cucumber, tofu, alfalfa and sesame seeds, dressed with Asian Dressing (see page 126 for recipe)

Black tahini slice (see page 118 for recipe)

Fruit leather (see page 96 recipe)

Apple & Nectarine

Popcorn, Macadamia nuts, Pumpkin seeds & Black rice biscuits

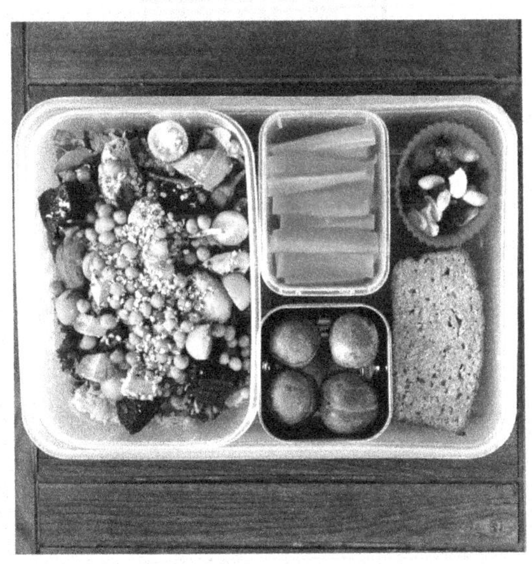

Straight from the tree

A Summer treat is always the abundance of fruit available, not only in the shops but also from our own trees. They don't all ripen at once, which is lovely as we get to appreciate each tree in turn. It begins with the apricots, then blood plums and finally peaches. Sometimes we have so many we remove the stones and freeze trays of fruit which we can use to make smoothies, even when the season has passed. Our home grown fruit is usually quite small, but what it lacks in size it definitely makes up for in flavour.

Salad of spinach, kale, brown rice, roasted squash, roasted beetroot, peas, home grown tomatoes, avocado and hemp seeds, dressed with balsamic vinegar

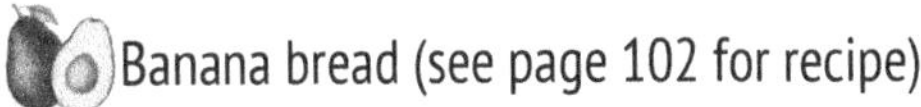

Banana bread (see page 102 for recipe)

Blood plums

Carrot sticks & Trail mix

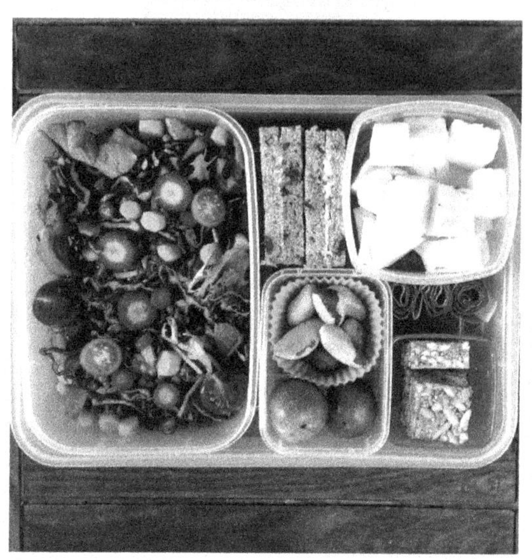

#nofilter

When selecting ingredients for lunchboxes, I am always drawn to colour. In my opinion, the best way to achieve that is by using fresh produce. You don't need anything artificial or an Instagram filter to have a lunch full of bright and beautiful colours. I remember making this salad and being so surprised when I cut into my purple carrot, only to discover its orange centre. I think it looks so beautiful.

- Salad of spinach, lentils, red cabbage, carrot, home grown lettuce and tomatoes, dressed with honey mustard dressing (see page 126 for recipe)

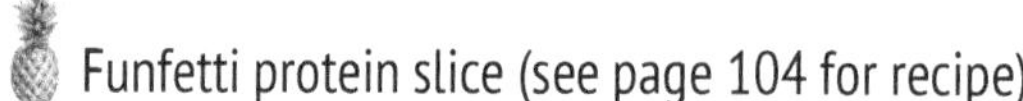

- Funfetti protein slice (see page 104 for recipe)
- Apricot fruit leather (see page 96 for recipe)
- Fruit loaf
- Blood plums & Pineapple
- Brazil nuts

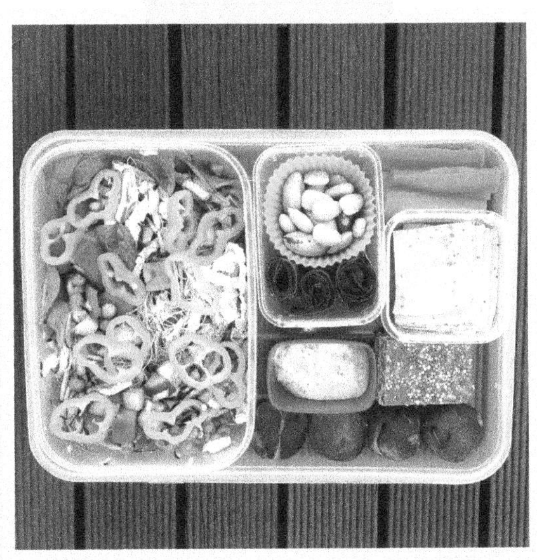

Sharing is caring

This is the time of year when everyone's veggie gardens and fruit trees are overflowing with produce - usually way too much for any one family. I might arrive home to find a bowl of tomatoes on my door step because somebody had too many. A friend could turn up with a bag of apricots or my neighbour will bring over veggies from her garden - and I'll share our produce too. It is such a lovely feeling of community. The zucchini in this salad is from a friend's garden and I am happy to reap the rewards of her bumper crop.

- Salad of spinach, Chinese cabbage, alfalfa, grated zucchini, cucumber, spring onion, peas, home grown tomatoes and capsicum, dressed with white balsamic vinegar
- Funfetti protein slice (see page 104 for recipe)
- Blood plum fruit leather (see page 96 for recipe)
- Home grown blood plums
- Mountain bread & Yogurt and herb dip
- Carrot sticks, Blanched almonds & Brazil nuts

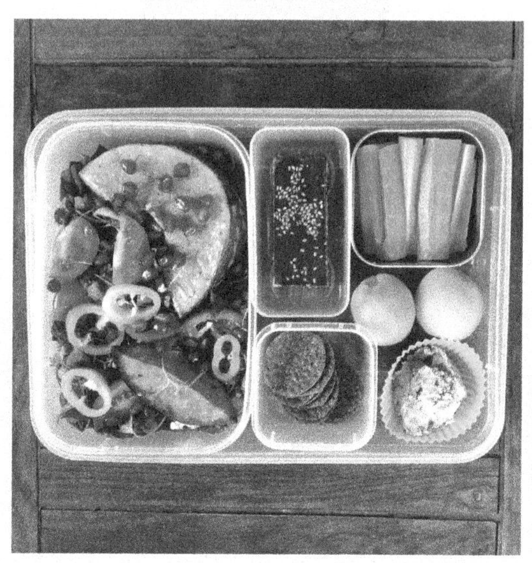

aubergine queen

The first time I planted eggplants - along with my other Summer vegetables - it went well. Very well actually. We may have only planted one pot but we had many, many mini eggplants. They were on the small side, I think they may have needed a bigger pot, but we still enjoyed them. Like in this dip. To make the dip I cut up a tray full of mini eggplants, drizzled them with olive oil and Himalayan salt and roasted them until soft. I then blitzed them with lemon juice, garlic and tahini.

- Salad of spinach, wombok, micro herbs, home grown tomatoes, capsicum, roast pumpkin and pomegranate, dressed with white balsamic vinegar
- 1 + 1 + 1 slice (see page 98 for recipe)
- Apricots
- Carrot sticks
- Black rice biscuits & Eggplant dip (see recipe in the subheading above)

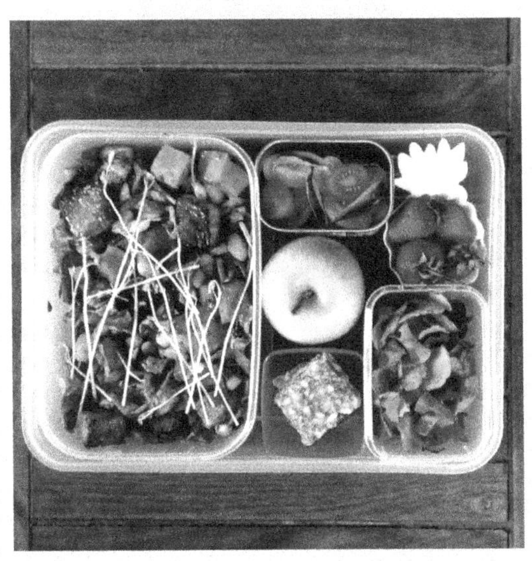

Back to school

In the weeks leading up to the start of the school year, the shops begin to stock their 'back to school' range. There are always so many containers, of all different shapes and sizes. I am hopeless and always end up buying more than I need. When I saw these fruit shaped silicone cups, I just had to have them. I still use them too, even to pack in my grown-up-husband's lunch box.

- Salad of rainbow chard, spinach, purple cabbage, white beans, roast pumpkin and snow pea sprouts, dressed with balsamic vinegar
- Bek's date and nut slice (see page 100 recipe)
- Apple & Strawberries
- Home grown tomatoes & Basil leaves
- Vegetable chips

Autumn

Both myself and my two sons celebrate birthdays in Autumn - so it is a time for celebration in my family. We also go away with friends to the high country for Easter each year. It's usually the first time I am getting my boots out, ready for some crisp mountain air. I love that in-between weather when fire restrictions are lifted so you can enjoy a campfire, but it's not too cold to sit around it all evening.

As the weather cools down, I start to crave more filling foods. I will begin to add additional ingredients to salads to make them more filling - like roast veggies or cheese. My son's favourite apples are Pink Ladies and I enjoy them too. I continually check in with the growers at the markets, asking them when they'll begin picking. They usually begin in April and I'm always excited to get my first bag for the season.

As well as apples, at this time of year you can enjoy figs, nectarines, pears, persimmons and quinces. Great Autumn veggies include beans, cucumbers, eggplants, potatoes, pumpkins, sweetcorn, turnips and zucchini.

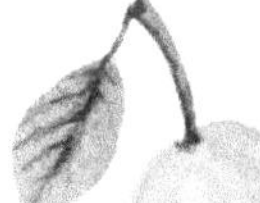
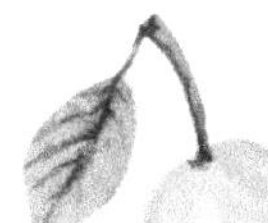

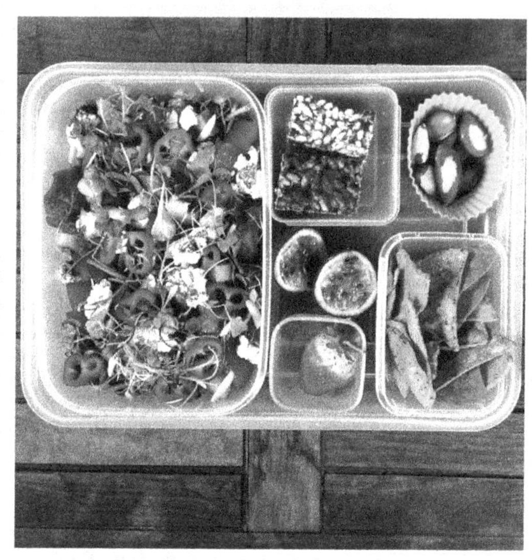

The last strawberry

The thing I love about this lunchbox ... is that strawberry. I remember I went out to water the garden, and there it was! One huge strawberry (and a few smaller green ones). I knew those little ones would not ripen now that the weather was beginning to cool. So for me, that strawberry said: 'Goodbye warm Summer days and hello Autumn!'

- Salad of spinach, cucumber, tomato, slivered almonds, capsicum, alfalfa, marinated Persian feta and salad herbs, dressed with white balsamic vinegar
- Choc-rice slice (see page 106 for recipe)
- Brazil nuts
- Corn chips
- Passionfruit & One last strawberry

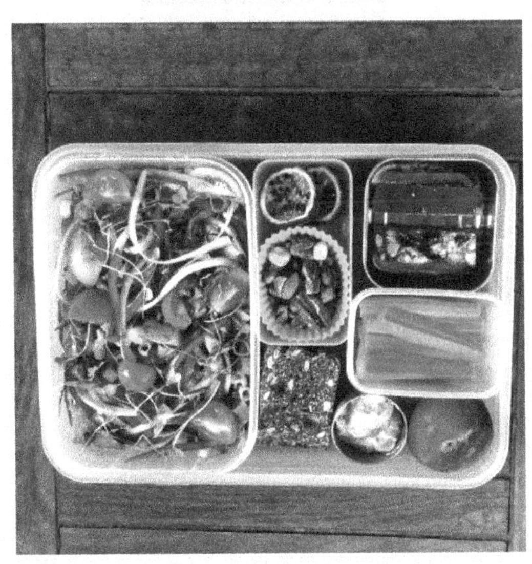

Pretty little greens

Usually when I am building a salad, I will start with a big handful of a leafy greens - and go from there. However, this crunchy slaw is a nice change of pace. There are many handy kitchen gadgets that make these types of salad a breeze to make. For this salad I've used a julienne peeler for my colourful carrot strips and a spiriliser for the zoodles.

- Salad of zoodles, Chinese cabbage, red cabbage, coloured carrot strips, spring onion, home grown tomato and salad herbs, dressed with white balsamic vinegar
- 1 + 1 + 1 slice (see page 98 for recipe)
- Carrot sticks & Hummus
- Pecan and rosemary crackers & Trail mix
- Plum & Passionfruit

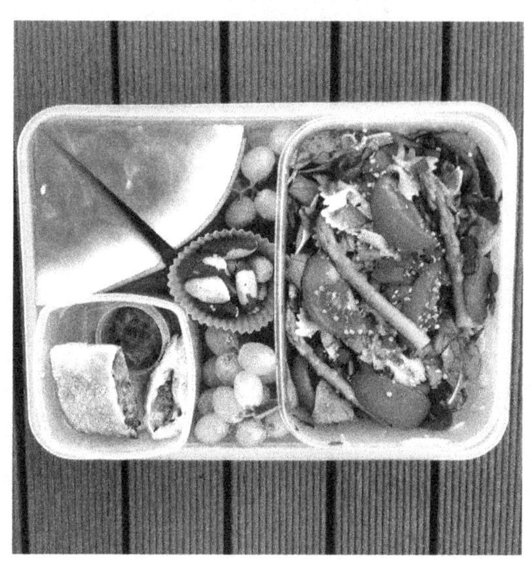

Snacks a-plenty

Having my fruit prepped can save me time in the midst of a hectic week. If I buy a large piece of watermelon or a pineapple, I usually chop it into pieces and store in several serving size containers. Or, I cut the watermelon into wedges, so it is easy to grab and pack. When I bring home a big bag of grapes, I wash them then use scissors to cut them into smaller bunches. I keep them in a bowl in the fridge so they can easily be grabbed as a snack or popped into a lunch box.

- Salad of spinach, pasta, capsicum, parsley, red onion, asparagus and hemp seeds, dressed with balsamic vinegar
- Veggie 'sausage' rolls (see page 82 for recipe) & Relish (see page 126 for recipe)
- Watermelon & Grapes
- Brazil nuts

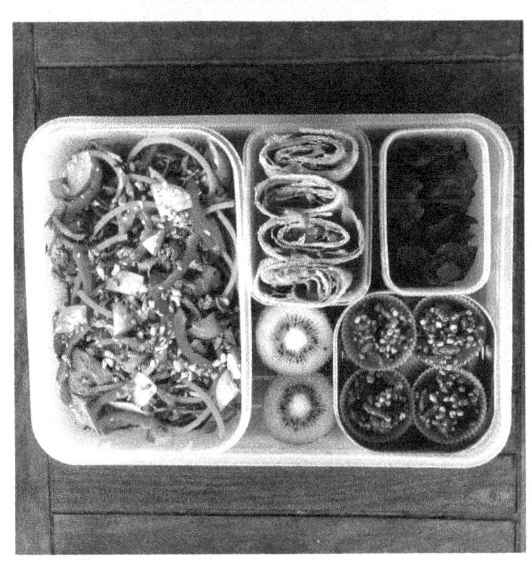

all wrapped up

Nearly every parent who has packed a lunch will have had that experience of finding it uneaten at the end of the day. Early on, I discovered that if I packed something that was going to take my boys a long time to eat – they wouldn't bother...it cut into valuable playing time! Snacks that can be eaten on the go are a great addition to lunch boxes - for both young and old. Wraps are a winner in our household and I love to get creative with different fillings.

- Salad of lettuce, mizuna, red cabbage, radish, red onion, carrot, capsicum, chopped almonds and sun flower seeds, with honey mustard dressing (see page 124 for recipe)

- Chocolate crackles (see page 108 for recipe)

- Kiwi fruit

- Beetroot chips

- Spinach wraps filled with beetroot tzatiki and fresh spinach

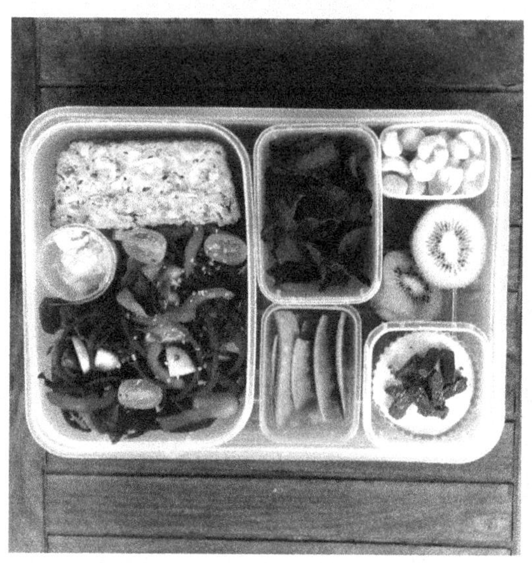

Going nuts

The first time I made nut loaf it was for Christmas dinner with my extended family. Everyone else was going to be enjoying traditional Christmas food and I wanted something festive I could enjoy too. Since then I have been a total nut loaf fan and make it regularly. It is filling and full of umami flavour. It is great served warm or cold, making it perfect to pack in lunch boxes.

- Salad of spinach, cucumber, purple carrot and tomatoes, served with a slice of nut loaf (see page 84 for recipe) and cashew cheese, dressed with white balsamic vinegar
- Raw fig 'cheesecake' (see page 110 for recipe)
- Kiwi fruit & Cashews
- Beetroot chips & Snow peas

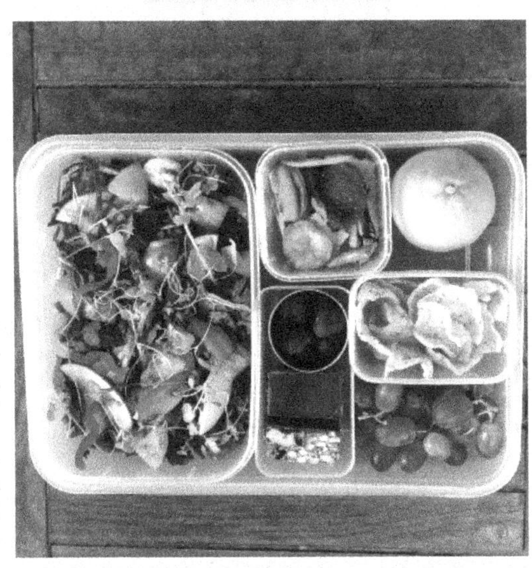

Autumn is for apples

As the season changes, so do the choices in fruit. When it is finally time to say goodbye to stone fruit, I buy mandarins, raspberries, red grapes and crisp crunchy apples from Harcourt. My youngest loves Pink Lady apples and at this time of the year they are at their very best. My apple and red cabbage salad with honey mustard dressing is a family favourite and is a great way to celebrate this beautiful fruit.

- Salad of lettuce, Chinese cabbage, red cabbage, home grown tomatoes, apples, capsicum and micro herbs, dressed with honey mustard dressing (see page 126 for recipe)

- 1 + 1 + 1 slice (see page 98 for recipe)

- Mandarin & Crimson grapes

- Vegetable chips & Chia crisps

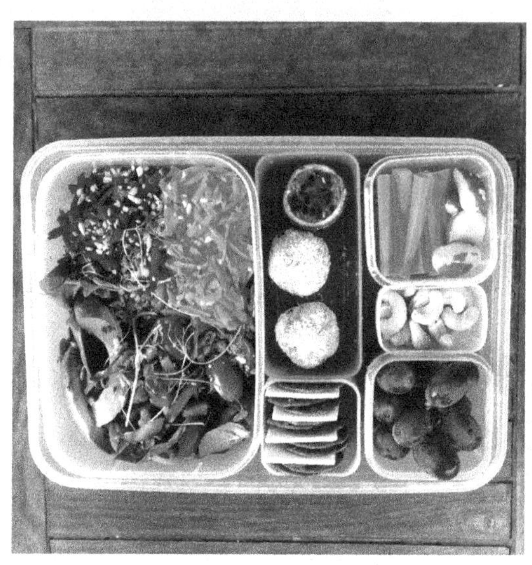

Food snaps

My favourite place to take food photos is at the front of our house. We have a bench seat under our verandah and the light there throughout the day is lovely. What you can't see is that I often have an audience. My cat and dog both like to run to the window for my 'food shoots' and watch with interest. I've tried time and time again to snap a picture of them to share but as soon as I move they run back to the door to greet me on my way back in. It always makes me smile.

- Salad of spinach, rocket, tomato, micro herbs, avocado, capsicum, carrot, beetroot and protein nut and seed mix, dressed with white balsamic vinegar
- Lemon meringue bliss balls (see page 114 for recipe)
- Passionfruit & Crimson grapes
- Carrot sticks & Brazil nuts and cashews
- Black rice biscuits, cheese and cucumber

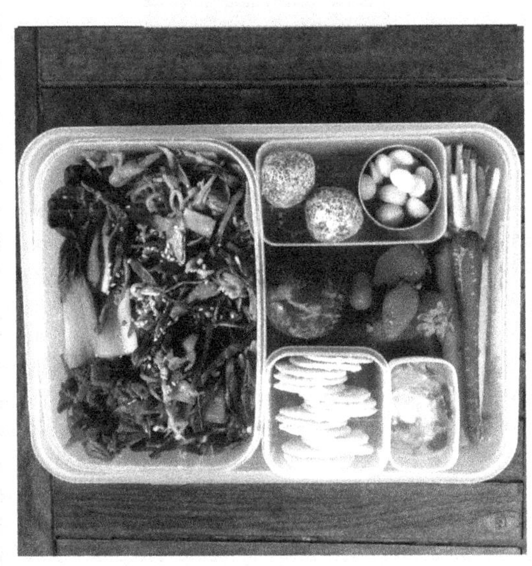

Jack in the box

It's always great to try new foods, but it even took me a little while to work up the courage to try this 'pulled pork' substitute made using canned jackfruit. I have cooked it a few times now and even the boys are on board with it as a tasty vegetarian meal option. The leftovers work well in a lunchbox, like in this noodle style salad.

- Salad of spinach, red cabbage, egg noodles, snow peas, sesame seeds, steamed bok choy and pulled jackfruit (see page 86 for recipe)
- Banoffee bliss balls (see page 116 for recipe)
- A Plum & Strawberries
- Carrots & Macadamias
- Rice crackers & Hummus dip

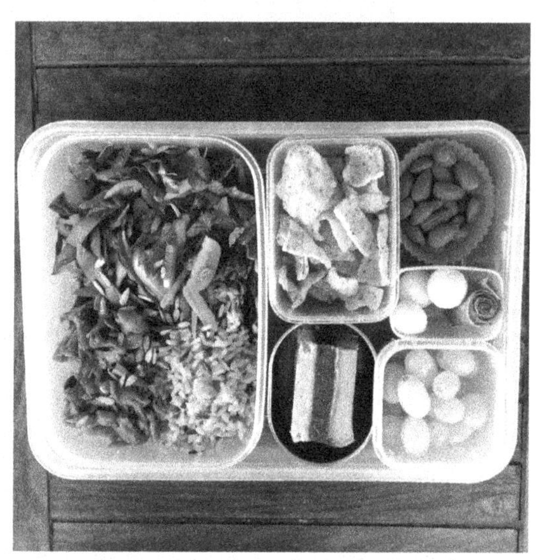

Well-rounded lunch

I like to have a variety of snacks in each lunchbox that I pack. This usually includes fresh fruit, a homemade treat and a few savoury options too; like nuts, crackers, chips and dip. There is such a wide variety of vegan dips and vegetable and legume chips available now and there always seems to be a new one to try. When selecting products I like to read the label and look for a short list of natural ingredients. I'm also drawn to what is new and interesting, or what is on special!

- Salad of spinach, cabbage, carrot, capsicum, and tomato with pulled jackfruit and wild rice, dressed with Asian dressing (see page 126 for recipe)

- Matcha slice (see page 120 for recipe)

- Apricot balls & Fruit leather (see page 96 for recipe)

- Grapes

- Chia crisps & Almonds

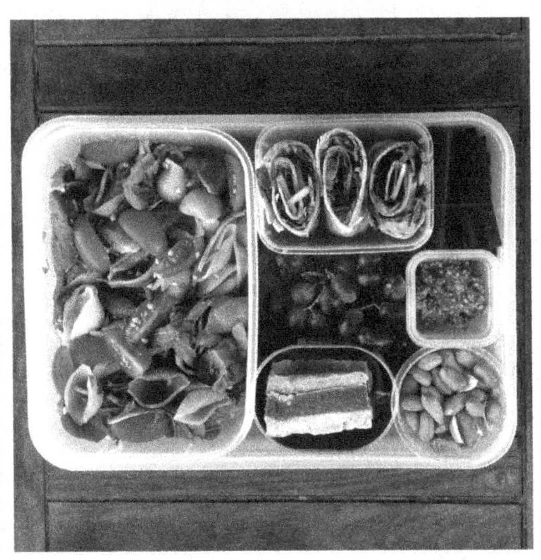

Hello pumpkin

Pumpkin seed oil is another beautiful product I buy at my local Farmers' Market. Made at an artisan oil mill, this pumpkin seed oil is known for having many health benefits. However, I buy it because of the beautiful taste. I don't eat a lot of pasta - but a little bit tossed in this oil is delicious. My youngest and I also love roast veggies and spaghetti drizzled with this oil. there is no need to include a dressing in this salad - the pumpkin seed oil does the job.

- Salad of pasta shells tossed in pumpkin seed oil with spinach, red cabbage, mizuna, tomato and hemp seeds

- Matcha slice (see page 120 for recipe)

- Wraps with beetroot tzatiki, spinach and radish

- Grapes

- Carrot sticks, Raw peanuts & Coriander dip

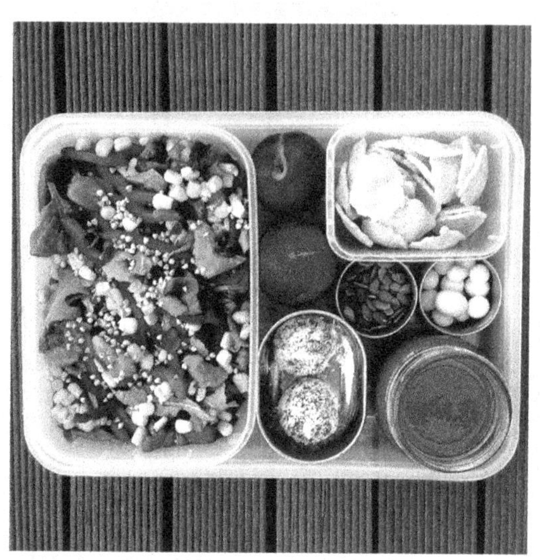

Beets me

I have a slight obsession with beetroot. I never used to like it at all - but that was when my only experience was with the canned variety. Now that I've discovered fresh beetroot, I absolutely love it. I use it to make juices. I grate it and add it to salads. I've used it to make cakes, felafel and vegetarian burgers. It is so versatile. However, this soup would have to be one of my favourite beetroot recipes. And as the weather cools down, packing a jar of soup helps our lunchboxes change with the season.

- Salad of lettuce, cabbage, roast pumpkin, raw grated beetroot, capsicum, corn and buckinis, dressed with white balsamic vinegar
- Banoffee bliss balls (see page 116 for recipe)
- Beetroot soup (see page 88 for recipe)
- Nectarines
- Veggie chips, Pumpkin seeds & Yogurt covered cranberries

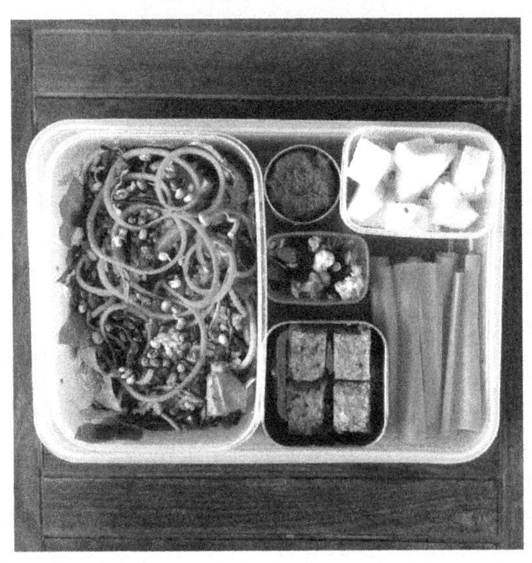

Winter is coming

There is always that one week in May, where the weather changes. When I stop holding out hope for an unexpected warm, sunny day. When the air is crisp and the mornings are frosty. When I can no longer deny that Winter is on its way. This is when I begin bulking out our salads. The addition of brown rice makes our salads a little more hearty, to keep us full and warm. Rice salads are also delicious with an Asian style dressing.

- Salad of brown rice, spinach, purple cabbage, red onion, yellow tomatoes, carrots and sprouts, dressed with Asian style dressing (see page 126 for recipe)
- Bek's date & nut slice (see page 100 for recipe)
- Pineapple
- Carrot sticks & Beetroot dip
- Trail mix

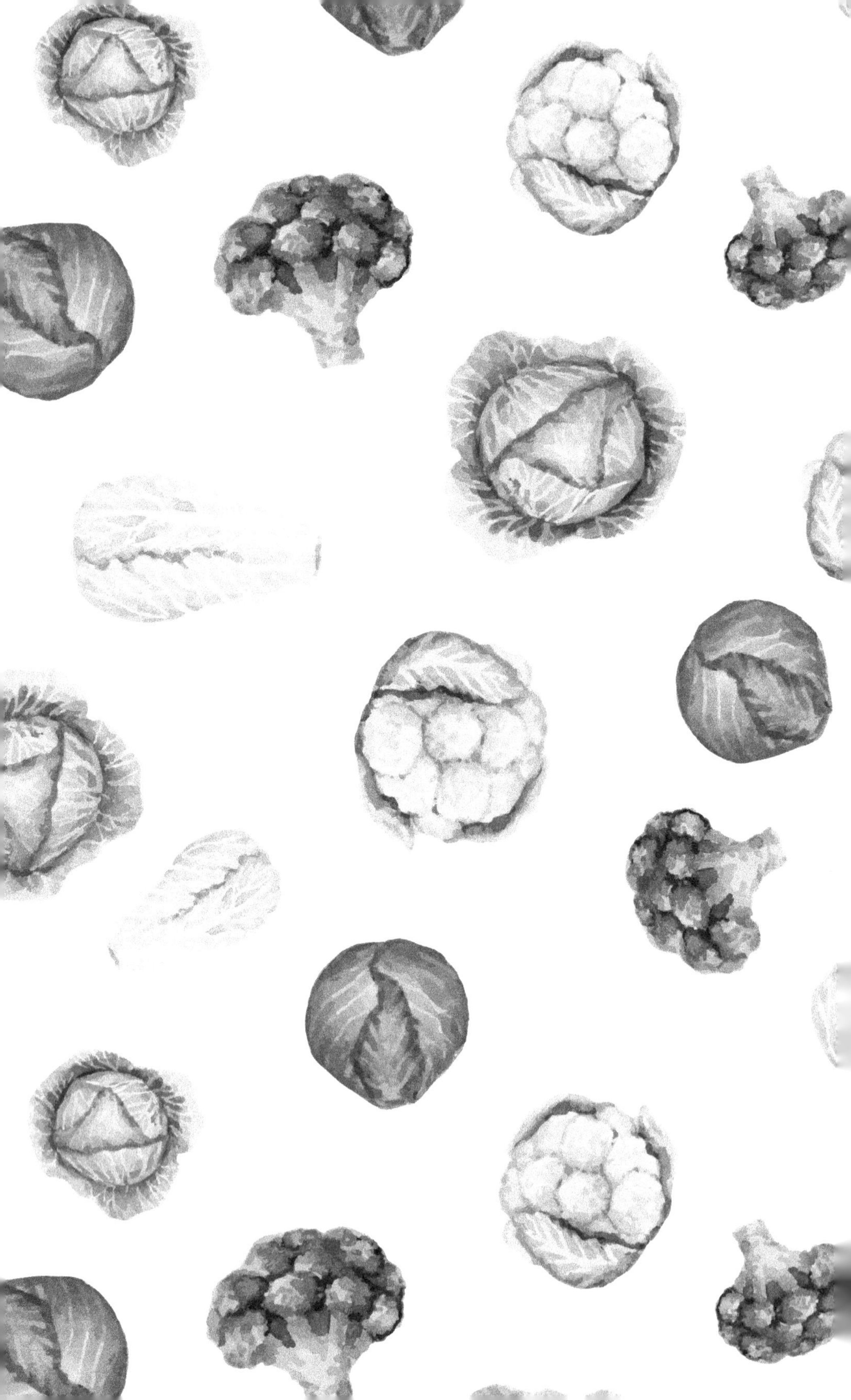

Winter

In Winter, I miss the sun, the daylight and the warmth, however I do love the chance to snuggle up inside on a rainy day - especially if there's a fire. I love to run in Winter. I never have to worry about overheating and I even love running in the rain. Cold days mean I often have the track all to myself. Winter clothes are great too - leggings, boots and coats - all so comfy and warm.

I crave large, warm filling meals during this time of year. I make vegetable curries, veggie lasagnes and lots of soup. I have found screw-top jars a great way to include soup in our lunches. I can tip it into a mug at work, heat it and carry it around with me. I add more carbs, like rice or pasta, to make salads more filling and I like to pack something that can be heated - like a slice of nut loaf.

When the weather is cool it is time to enjoy cabbage, brussels sprouts, pumpkin, potatoes, onions, beets, carrots, turnips, parsnips, sweet potato, kale, fennel, silverbeet, garlic, ginger, leeks, asian greens and avocado. For fruit, there's citrus fruit, pomegranates, rhubarb, pears, grapefruit and, as Winter ends, pineapple and paw paw.

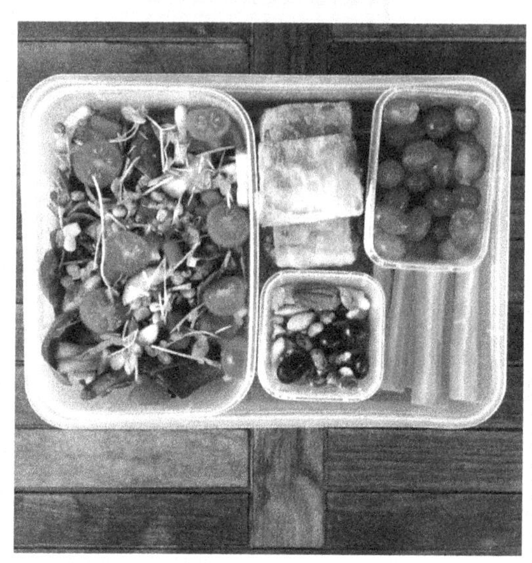

Heat me up

Whenever my brothers visit, my mum always bakes them her famous sausage rolls. She's been making these since we were little and as a child they were one of my favourites. Whenever I see and smell them, I can't help but reminisce and I really wanted to recreate that dish from my childhood - but a version I could now enjoy. These vegetarian friendly veggie 'sausage' rolls are a great addition to a Winter lunchbox to warm you up and keep you full.

- Salad of spinach, cucumber, corn, tomato, mung bean sprouts and snow pea sprouts, dressed with white balsamic vinegar
- Veggie 'sausage' rolls (see page 82 for recipe)
- Crimson grapes & Carrot sticks
- Trail mix

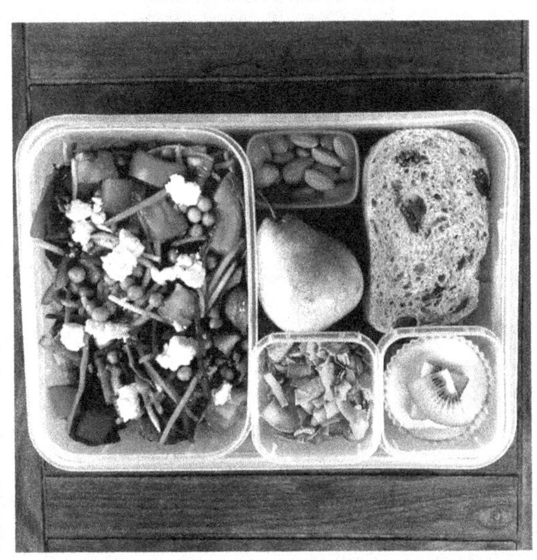

Warm & toasty

The smell of toast on a cold Winters' day is an instant pick-me-up. I love being able to enjoy that comforting Winter treat at work by packing a slice of bread to pop into the toaster. I don't eat a lot of bread, so when I do, I make sure it is a good quality slice that I know I'll really enjoy. This beautiful olive bread is from a local artisan bakery. Their fruit loaf is also featured in another of the Winter lunchboxes.

- Salad of spinach, carrot, broccoli stem, beetroot, peas, capsicum, tomato and goat's cheese, dressed with balsamic vinegar
- Raw fig 'cheesecake' topped with kiwi fruit (see page 110 for recipe)
- Pear
- Almonds & Coconut chips
- Olive bread

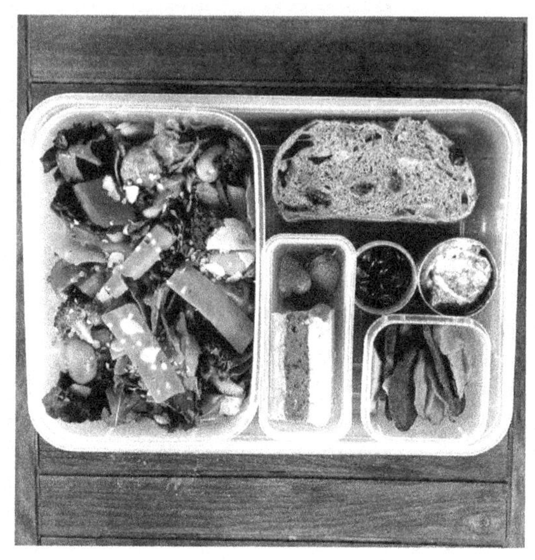

Steam away the blues

Sometimes when I'm feeling those Winter blues, I'll steam a big pot of veggies and devour a bowl full. It always makes me feel better and it's so comforting in the colder weather. The left overs are a great addition to a Winter salad. Although the boys and I like them, it is my husband who screws his nose up at brussels sprouts - he wasn't too pleased to find one had snuck into his salad this day!

- Salad of spinach, rocket, kale, butter beans, tomato, hemp seeds, flaked almonds and left over steamed vegetables: brussels sprouts, carrots and capsicum (can be warmed if you like)

- Strawberries & Matcha slice (see page 120 for recipe)

- Walnut and raisin loaf

- Vegetable chips & Kale and white bean dip

- Chocolate covered pumpkin seeds

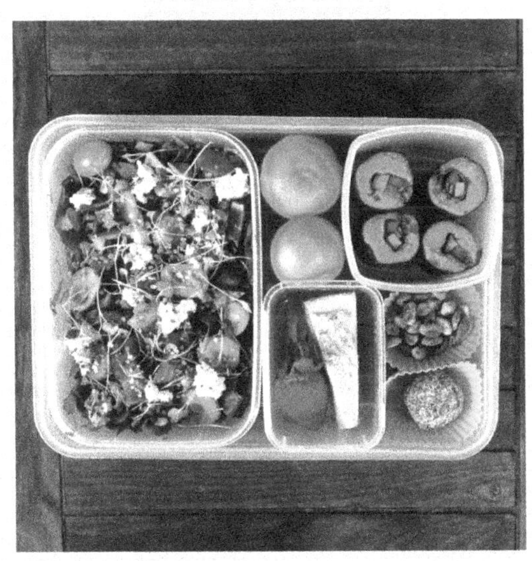

Sweet, sweet sushi

Sweet potato sushi is a great way to use up leftover mash and put an extra serving of veggies into a lunchbox. I always add miso paste to the leftover sweet potato mash to give it a flavour boost. Then fill and roll as you would ordinary sushi. Be warned, it can get a little messy making these - but the end product is worth it.

- Salad of rainbow chard, spinach, micro herbs, carrot, tomatoes, goat's cheese and hemp seeds, dressed with white balsamic vinegar
- Raw fig 'cheesecake' (see page 110 for recipe)
- Banoffee bliss ball (see page 116 for recipe)
- Sweet potato sushi
- Mandarins, Strawberry & Pistachios

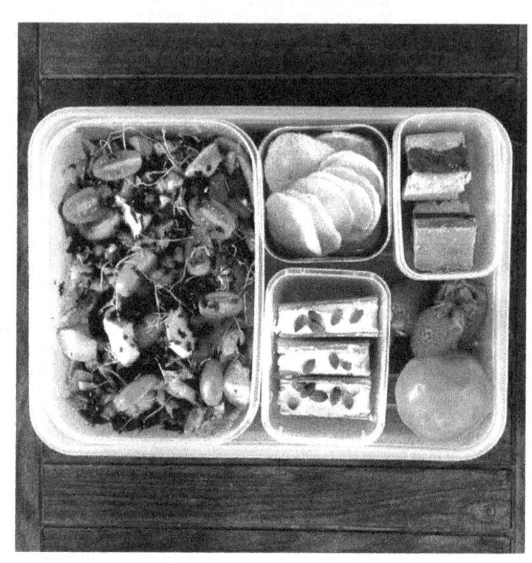

In a pickle

I am officially on the bandwagon of fermented foods. I usually have a bottle of kombucha in my fridge as well as a jar of kraut. I know many people make their own fermented foods, but currently I just buy mine from the whole foods store. The main reason I include these foods in my diet is to improve the balance of good bacteria in the gut. Adding kraut to salads is a great way to include fermented foods in your diet.

- Salad of spinach, sauerkraut, peas, capsicum, tomato, avocado and sea weed flakes, dressed with white balsamic vinegar
- Matcha slice (see page 120 for recipe)
- Mandarin & Strawberries
- Veggie chips
- Celery with cream cheese and pumpkin seeds

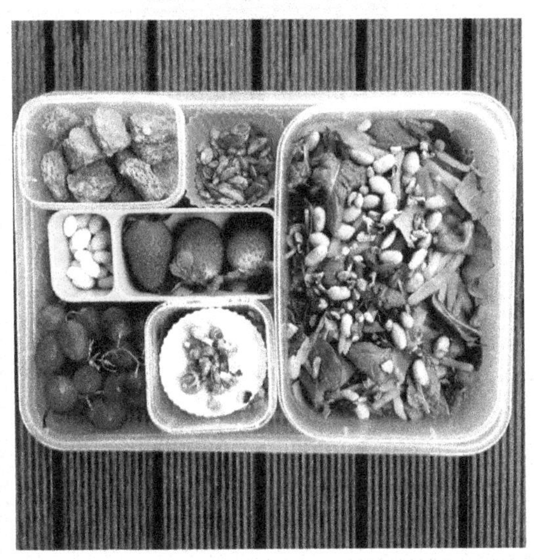

So cool

You may not always think to look in your freezer for salad ingredients, but I regularly use frozen peas, corn and beans in my salads, like these edamame beans. If I am photographing a lunchbox or eating a salad straight away, I'll blanch them in a little boiling water for a minute or two. However, if I am packing lunches ahead of time, I will just add them to our salads frozen, they will thaw by the time the salad is ready to eat.

- Salad of brown rice, spinach, red cabbage, capsicum, grated carrot, edamame beans and walnuts, dressed with Asian dressing (see page 126 for recipe)
- Raw fig 'cheesecake' (see page 112 for recipe) topped with pistachios
- Strawberries & Crimson grapes
- Yogurt covered goji berries & Lime chilli seed mix
- Mini weet bix

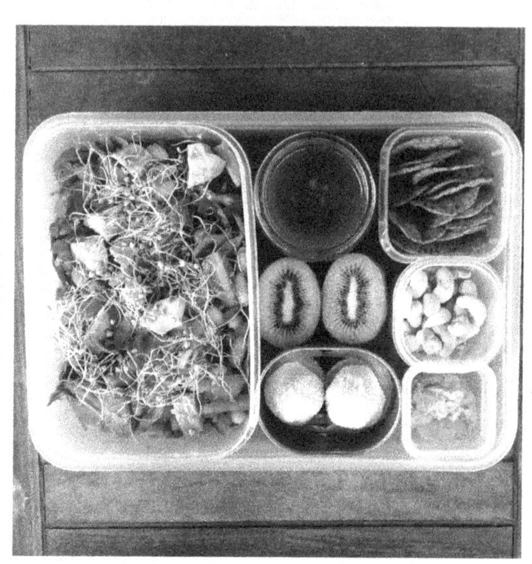

Pure bliss

Bliss balls are such an easy and healthy snack to make. There are so many different recipes and flavour combinations around now, you are sure to find one you'll love. If not, get creative - there are no real rules when making bliss balls, which is my favourite way to cook! Too dry? Add more honey or coconut oil or tahini. Too wet? Add oats, almond meal or coconut. These Lemon Meringue bliss balls are one of my all-time favourite flavours, you will find the recipe on page 114.

- Salad of spinach, cannellini beans, red cabbage, capsicum, tomato, avocado, alfalfa and buckinis, dressed with white balsamic vinegar
- Beetroot soup (see page 88 for recipe)
- Lemon meringue bliss balls (see page 114 for recipe)
- Kiwi fruit & Cashews
- Felafel crisps & Carrot dip

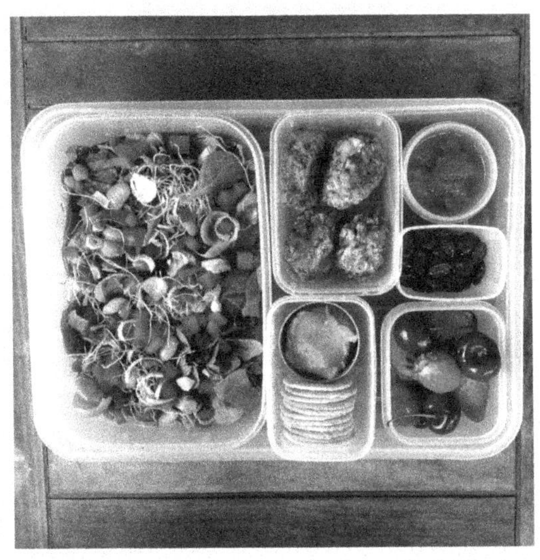

Magic of mushrooms

When I was young, I remember my mum's layered salad was always popular at Christmas. It included a layer of raw mushrooms - which I always thought was an odd choice, but it was something I enjoyed. There are actually many vegetables I enjoy raw - and not the ones you may typically think of. Often as I am cutting up vegetables for dinner, I'll snack on raw broccoli or cauliflower, and this salad includes both raw mushrooms and brussels sprouts. Maybe that's why whatever the weather, I love including salads in our lunches.

- Salad of 4 bean mix, spinach, mushroom, alfalfa, capsicum and Baby Brussel sprouts, dressed with white balsamic vinegar
- Broccoli nuggets with relish (see page 90 for recipe)
- Strawberries and cherries
- Brown rice crackers & Carrot dip
- Pumpkin seeds coated in dark chocolate

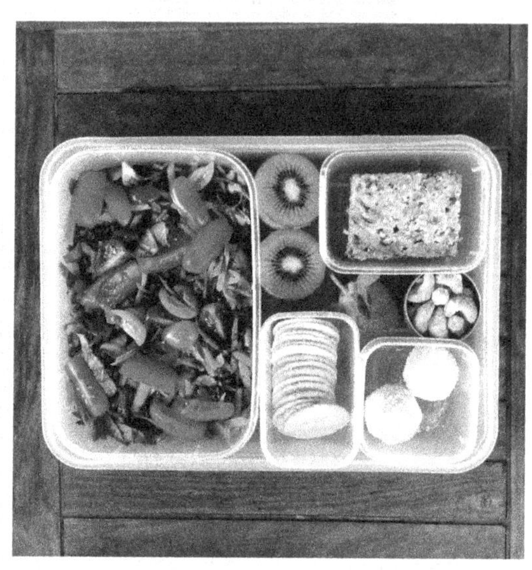

Nice as rice

Salads made with rice as the base are great to heat up on a cold day and adding rice is also a great way to bulk a salad up for Winter. There are many varieties of rice so it is worth exploring the choices available. This salad features black rice, often referred to as 'the forbidden rice' - which always seems to make me want it even more! Not only that, black rice is high in protein, fibre and iron so it's a great nutritional boost too.

- Salad of black rice, spinach, grated carrot, tomato, dressed with Asian dressing (see page 126 for recipe)
- Nut loaf (see page 84 for recipe)
- Lemon meringue bliss balls (see page 114 for recipe)
- Kiwi fruit & Strawberry
- Brown rice crackers & Honey cashews

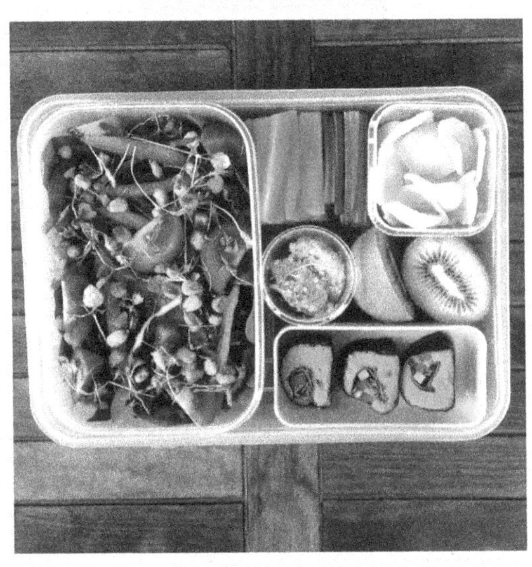

Old favourites

Veggie sticks are a staple lunch box snack. Sometimes we go through 3 bags of carrots in a week with the amount of carrot sticks I pack! While carrot sticks are the firm favourite - there are lots of other colourful options: celery, snow peas, capsicum, broccoli stem and rainbow chard all make occasional appearances in our lunches too. They all go perfectly with a little pot of your favourite dip.

- Salad of spinach, red cabbage, capsicum, tomato, micro herbs and crunchy corn kernels, dressed with white balsamic vinegar
- Sweet potato sushi (see page 57 for details)
- Kiwi fruit
- Vegetable sticks, Veggie chips & Vegan pumpkin and basil dip

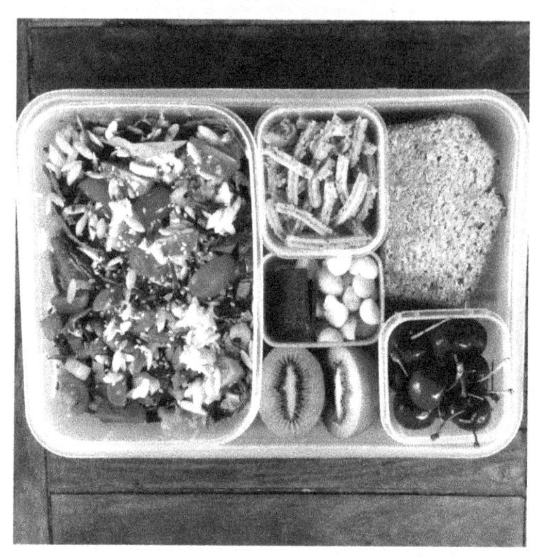

Going bananas

Bananas are another food I need to buy in bulk. In addition to packing them fresh in lunches or adding them to our muesli, we also freeze slices of banana so they can be thrown into smoothies. My eldest has a banana, cacao and almond milk smoothie for breakfast every morning. Of course they are also a wonderful ingredient when baking, as you will see in my banana bread recipe. A slice is perfect to eat as it is, or warm it up for a toasty Winter treat.

- Salad of risoni pasta, spinach, celery, tomato, purple cabbage and nut protein mix, dressed with white balsamic vinegar

- Banana bread (see page 102 for recipe)

- Kiwi fruit & Cherries

- Quinoa sticks

- Macadamia nuts and Dark chocolate

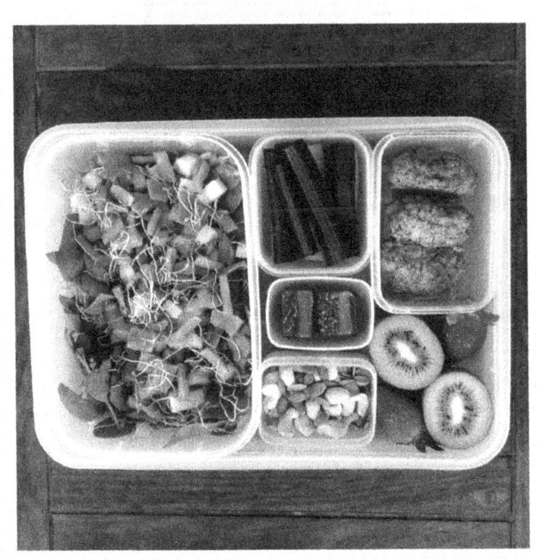

Keen on quinoa

Years ago, when quinoa was the new superfood on the block, I was keen to jump on the bandwagon. I made a quinoa risotto and proudly dished it up. My kids immediately started complaining and my response was: "it's a super food, it's an ancient grain, it's good for you!" which, of course, didn't impress them at all. I sat down to eat it, and they were right - it was awful! Years on, I've greatly improved my quinoa cooking abilities and it's a great addition to salads. My kids though, are still to be convinced!

- Salad of spinach, rice, quinoa, alfalfa, snow peas, capsicum and daikon radish, dressed with white balsamic vinegar
- Broccoli Nuggets (see page 90 for recipe)
- Peanut brittle fudge slice (see page 122 for recipe)
- Kiwi and strawberries
- Carrot sticks & Cashews and pumpkin seeds

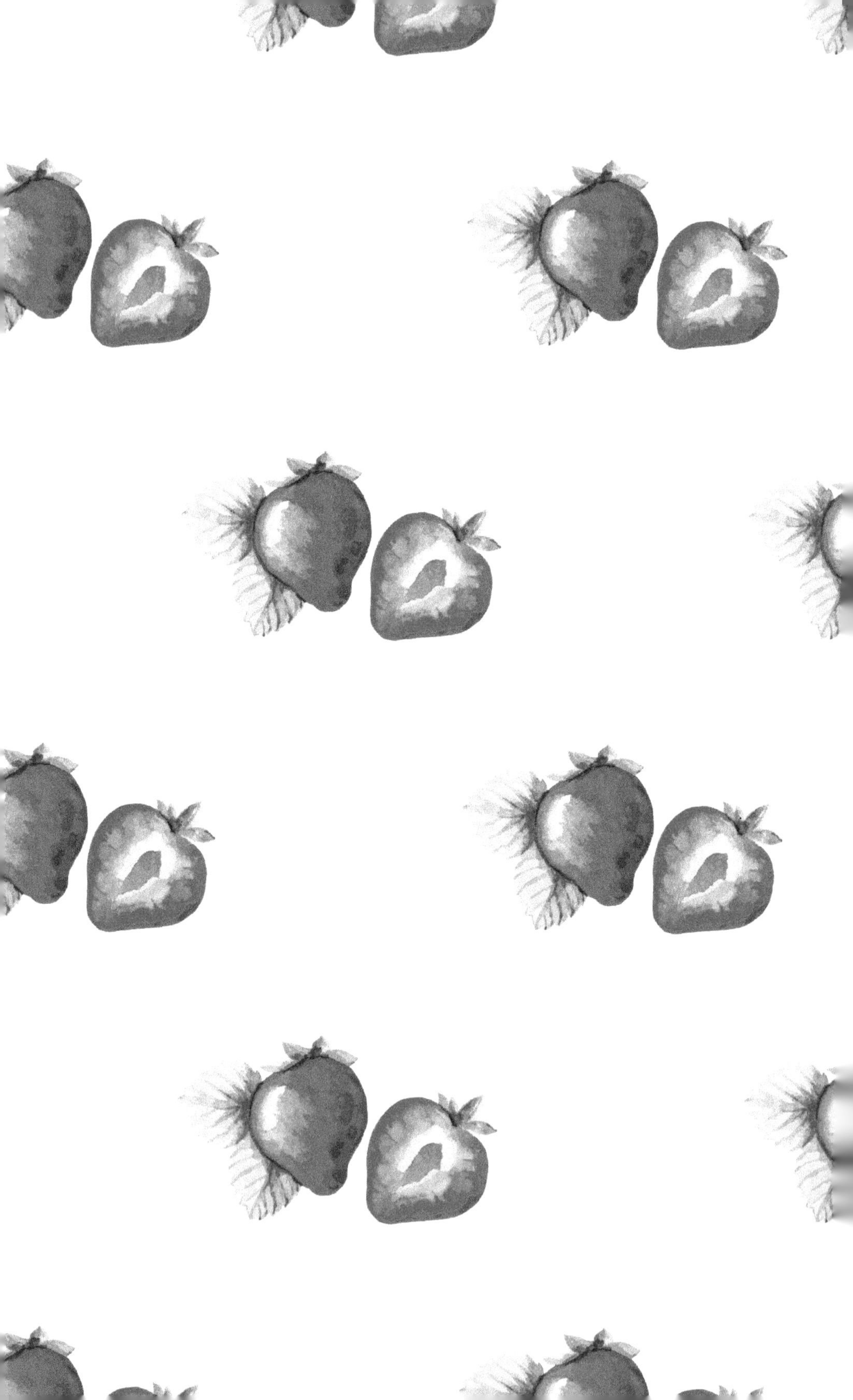

Spring

I love the smell of Spring. When I take the dog for a run, I can smell the flowers in bloom. I am lucky to live near bushland tracks where I can see birds, butterflies and other signs the season is changing. I am always super excited about daylight savings and the warmer weather makes me feel like I am coming out of hibernation.

In Spring, the first of the Summer fruits will appear in the stores - but they cost a fortune! I have innocently taken a bag of grapes to the counter, only to find them so expensive I needed to put them back! However, the mere sight of them has me craving peaches, plums and nectarines and the fruit content in our lunchboxes goes up!

This time of year is the perfect time to enjoy citrus fruits such as oranges, lemons and grapefruit as well as the first of the Summer seasons' fruit like strawberries and other berries. Check out Spring veggies such as artichokes, brussels sprouts, silverbeet, fennel and peas.

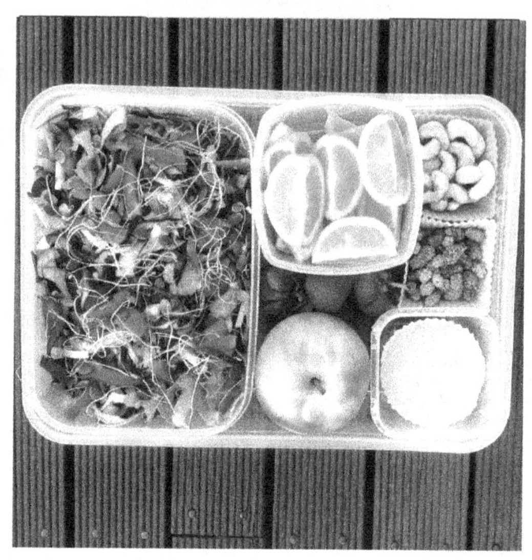

Spring zing

In Summer we enjoy our stone fruit trees, in Spring it is our citrus trees. We have a lemon, lime and two orange trees. My husband and my youngest love our oranges - I think their record is eating 12 in one day. Packing oranges whole can make them difficult to eat at school or work, so I prep them by cutting them into segments.

- Salad of iceberg lettuce, spinach, kale sprouts, purple cabbage, red capsicum, alfalfa and pumpkin seeds, dressed with white balsamic vinegar
- Raw mandarin 'cheesecake' (see page 112 for recipe)
- Apple, Strawberries & Home grown orange segments
- Cashews & White mulberries

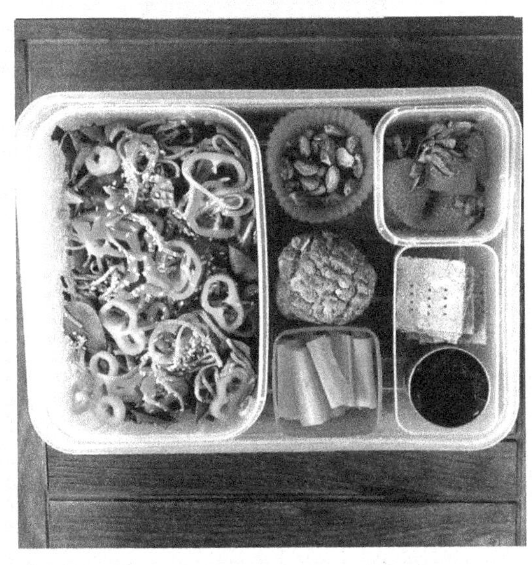

Snack in a cup

Silicone baking cups are a great addition to your lunch box container collection, they are so handy. I regularly use them when baking as you will see in the recipe section of this book. However, they are great when packing lunches too. If you are packing biscuits and want to serve an accompanying dip in the same container, the cup will keep it separate. They are also perfect for little servings of snacks such as nuts, seeds or dried fruit.

- Salad of spinach, lettuce, red cabbage, green tea noodles, capsicum and sesame seeds, dressed with Asian dressing (see page 126 for recipe)

- Herby chickpea crackers (see page 92 for recipe) with Beetroot relish (see page 126 for recipe)

- Strawberries

- Carrot sticks & Pistachios

- Coconut cookies

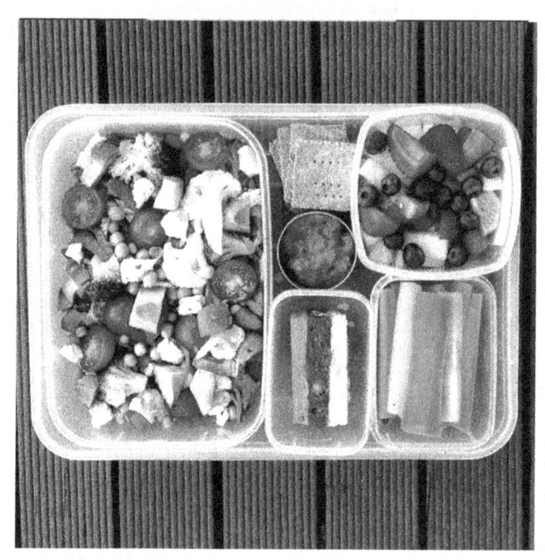

Sweet pea memory

My Nana and Poppy had the most beautiful vegetable garden. They grew so many different vegetables – including peas. When we were young, my brothers and I would pick, shell and eat fresh peas - the taste was amazing. It has brought back so many memories having tendrils of peas climbing through my Springtime garden and I've loved watching my children enjoy them too. However, the crop from my one little pot was devoured in less than a week!

- Salad of spinach, lettuce, brussels sprouts, freshly shelled peas, avocado, tomato, goat's cheese and steamed broccoli and cauliflower, dressed with white balsamic vinegar
- Matcha slice (see page 120 for recipe)
- Herby chickpea crackers (see page 92 for recipe)
- Fruit salad (pineapple, strawberries, kiwi and blue berries)
- Carrot sticks and broccoli stems & Ajvar (paprika relish)

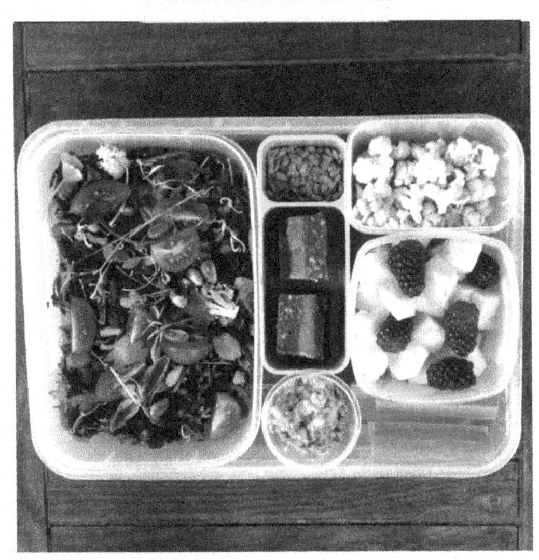

Travel for the palate

When I am at the Farmers' Market as soon as I see a new fruit or vegetable - I have to buy it and try it. In this case it was a beautiful green bunch of mizuna. I have since learned that mizuna is a Japanese salad ingredient with a peppery taste. It makes a lovely addition to salads, like this one.

- Salad of mizuna, spinach, rocket, grated beetroot, lentil sprouts, corn, tomato, broccoli and tomatoes, dressed with white balsamic vinegar
- Peanut brittle fudge slice (see page 122 for recipe)
- Pineapple & Crimson blackberries
- Carrot sticks & Kale and white bean dip
- Popcorn & Sunflower seeds

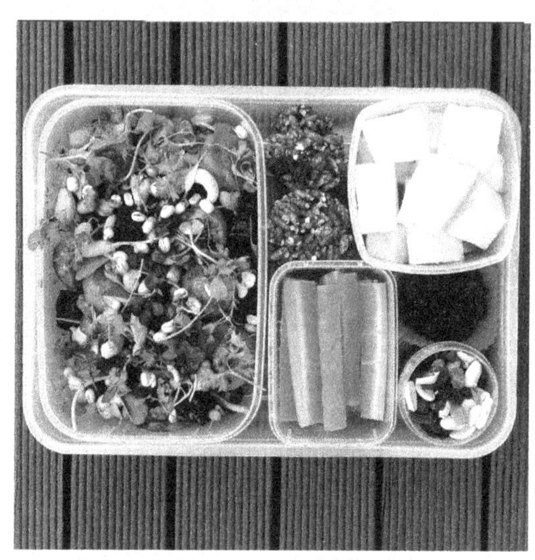

Roast of the day

A regular part of my Sunday preparation is to roast a large tray of vegetables. Sometimes it is to clean out my vegetable drawer - or sometimes it's because I've gone a little overboard at the Farmers' Market. I find it really convenient having these on hand. I can use them as the base of a quick vegetarian meal for myself through the week or as a salad ingredient, as shown in this lunchbox.

- Salad of spinach, roasted sweet potato, roasted beetroot, micro herbs, mung bean sprouts, edamame beans and cashews, dressed with balsamic vinegar
- Chocolate crackles (see page 108 for recipe)
- Pineapple
- Carrot sticks & Trail mix
- Beetroot relish (see page 126 for recipe)

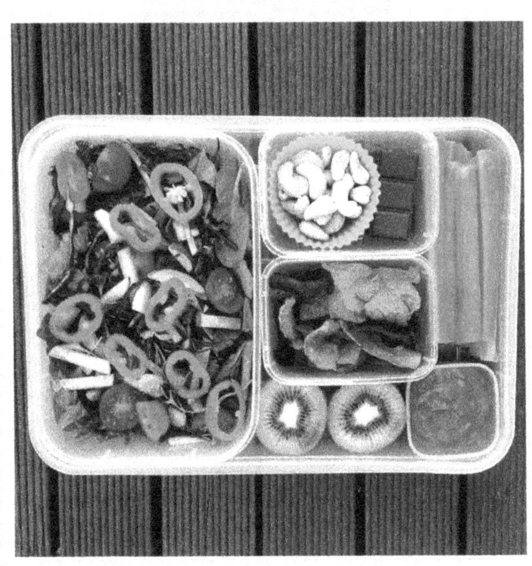

Packing tips

Packing these lunchboxes is sometimes like a game of Tetris - trying to get lunch and enough snacks for the day to all fit in perfectly. When I am putting lunches together I will tip things out and swap containers or try different types of fruit to see which one looks and fits the best. My family often give me strange looks, but they leave me to it - especially as they then directly benefit from my lunchbox arranging game.

- Salad of rainbow chard, spinach, micro herbs, radishes, cherry tomatoes, purple cabbage and capsicum, dressed with white balsamic vinegar
- Kiwi fruit
- Carrot sticks, Vegetable chips & Salsa dip
- Cashews & Cacao chocolate

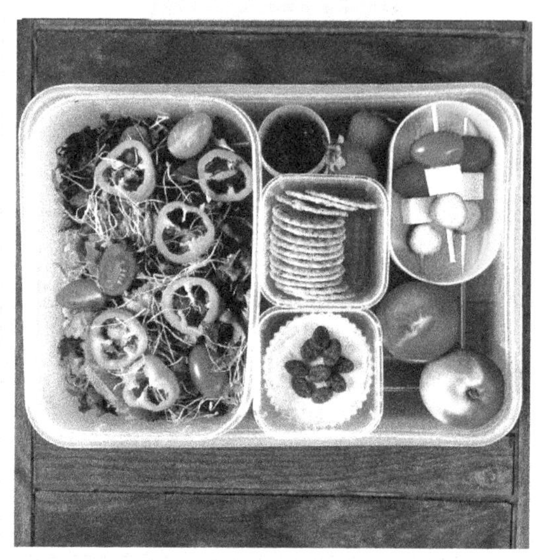

Fruit, glorious fruit

Hubby regularly drives around the Victorian countryside for work including through many fruit growing regions. He often returns home with boxes of fruit and these beautiful nectarines were our first for the season. I absolutely adore stone fruit, so I was beyond excited to see this locally grown produce. For me, it is also a sign that Summer, my favourite season, is on its way.

- Salad of brown rice, spinach, red kale, salad herbs, alfalfa, tomato and capsicum, dressed with Honey mustard dressing (see page 126 for recipe)
- Raw mandarin 'cheesecake' topped with choc-covered pumpkin seeds (see page 112 for recipe)
- Nectarines & Strawberries
- Brown rice crackers & Beetroot relish (see page 126 for recipe)
- Baby cucumber, tomato and cheese kebabs

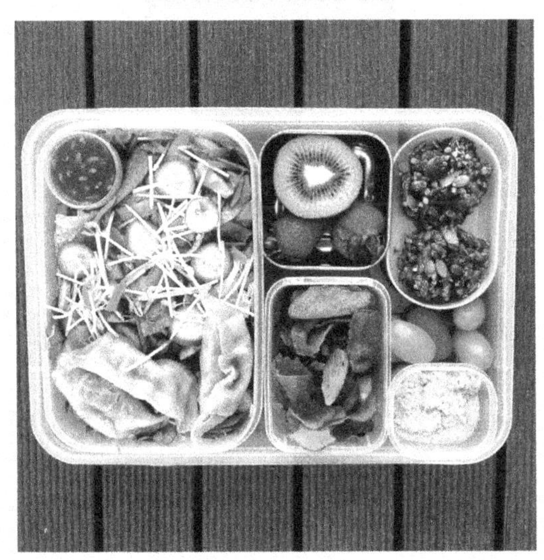

a dressy salad

One of the my most frequently asked questions on Instagram is, 'what do you use to dress your salads?' In each lunch I pack, I include a little pot similar to the one shown here. This way, we can pour the dressing over the salad when we eat, so the salad doesn't go soggy. Most of the time I pack balsamic vinegar, either white or red. But every now and again I get a bit fancy. The recipe for this Asian style dressing can be found on page 126.

- Gyoza with a salad of Chinese cabbage, carrot, cucumber, celery, snow peas and snow pea sprouts, dressed with Asian style dressing (see page 126 for recipe)

- Chocolate crackles (see page 108 recipe)

- Strawberries & Kiwi fruit

- Pumpkin and basil dip, Vegetable chips & Cherry tomatoes

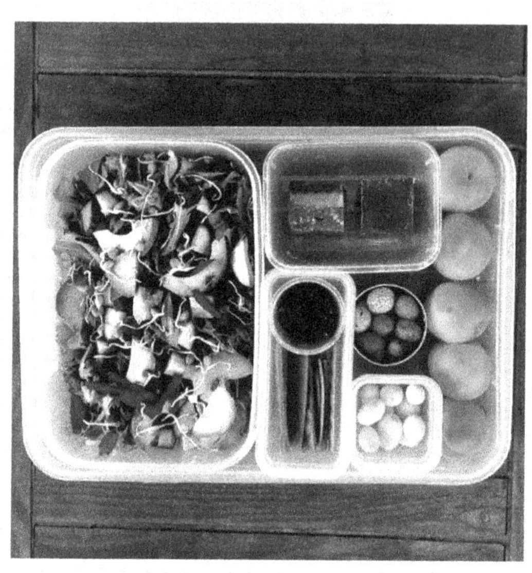

Furry fruit

One day my husband returned home with three boxes of beautiful stone fruit. We had so many, I decided to take a bag to school to share with my class. Some of my students had never seen or heard of apricots, peaches or nectarines. They thought it was hilarious that their fruit had fur and kept patting it, asking if they could eat these furry things? Some also asked about the spots. I explained that fruit directly from the farmer was a little different to the 'pretty' supermarket fruit - and tastier. It was lovely to see them enjoying beautiful, local produce and the whole bag had disappeared before recess.

- Salad of mizuna, cabbage, micro herbs, grated beetroot, lentil sprouts and avocado, dressed with white balsamic vinegar

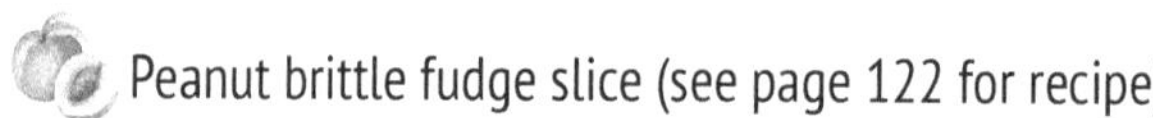

- Peanut brittle fudge slice (see page 122 for recipe)
- Kri Kri (covered peanuts) & Yogurt covered cranberries
- Snow peas & Beetroot relish
- Apricots

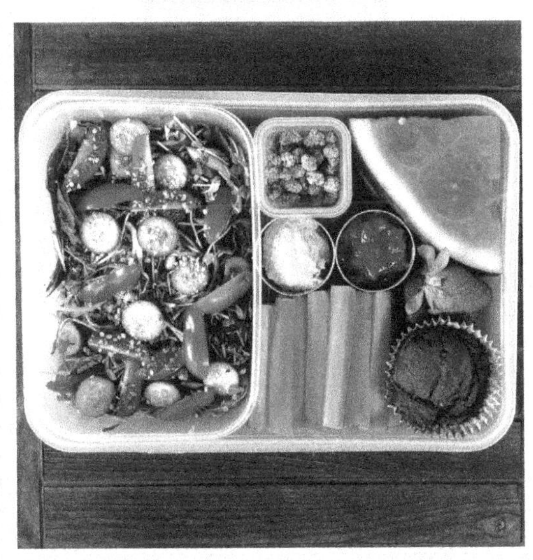

Loving leftovers

One of my pet hates is almost-empty jars or packets in my fridge or pantry - but this can be a blessing when packing small snacks for lunches. For example, there always seems to be an open jar of salsa in the fridge. I've found this can be used as a dip with veggie sticks or corn chips. Packets with only a small amount of seeds can be combined to make little snack pots...like this one with the white mulberries. Lunch boxes are a great way to use up leftover food rather than being wasteful.

- Salad of spinach, red cabbage, cucumber, snow pea sprouts, mung bean sprouts, carrot and tomato, dressed with white balsamic vinegar

- 12 Health Cacao protein muffin

- Watermelon & Strawberries

- White mulberries

- Carrot sticks, Salsa & Semi-dried tomato hummus

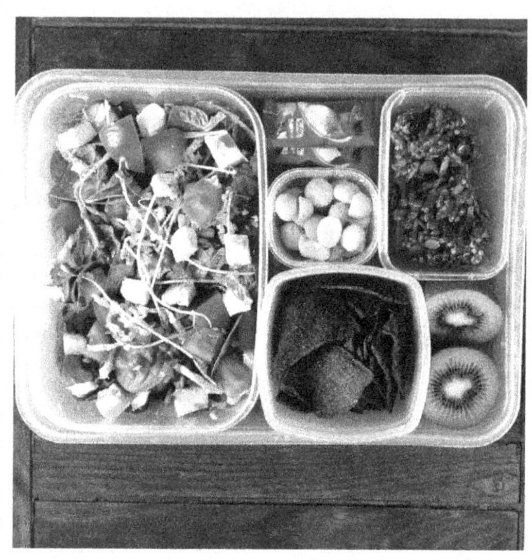

From the patch

Sometimes the random finds my husband brings home are awesome - like the time he came home with five kilograms of freshly picked apricots. Other times they're a bit odd, like the time he came home with a goat (don't worry, Stella is living happily on a friend's farm after I said no to her staying in our yard!) Then there was the time he came home from a visit with a friend at their market garden with the biggest cabbage I have ever seen, it was twice the size of my head! Needless to say, there were many cabbage dishes on the menu this week.

- Salad of cabbage, spinach, micro herbs, tomato, mung beans, snow pea sprouts and almond and apricot cream cheese, dressed with white balsamic vinegar
- Chocolate crackles (see page 108 for recipe)
- Kiwi fruit
- Nougat & Macadamia nuts
- Blue corn chips

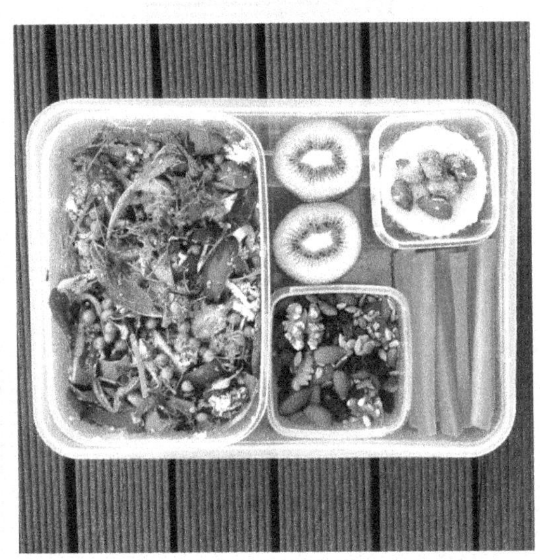

What a dill

Fresh herbs are amazing in salads. Herbs from my garden that I've used in salads include parsley, basil, coriander, mint and chives. They all have such distinct tastes and are a great way to add extra flavour to a salad. This salad features one of my favourite herbs, dill. The smell and the taste remind me of my Nana's cooking. It is amazing how the sense of smell can evoke such strong memories - even from back when you were young.

- Salad of couscous, spinach, carrot, red cabbage, cucumber, tomato, Persian feta and dill, dressed with white balsamic vinegar
- Raw mandarin 'cheesecake' (see page 112 for recipe) topped with sugared almonds
- Kiwi fruit
- Trail mix & Carrot sticks

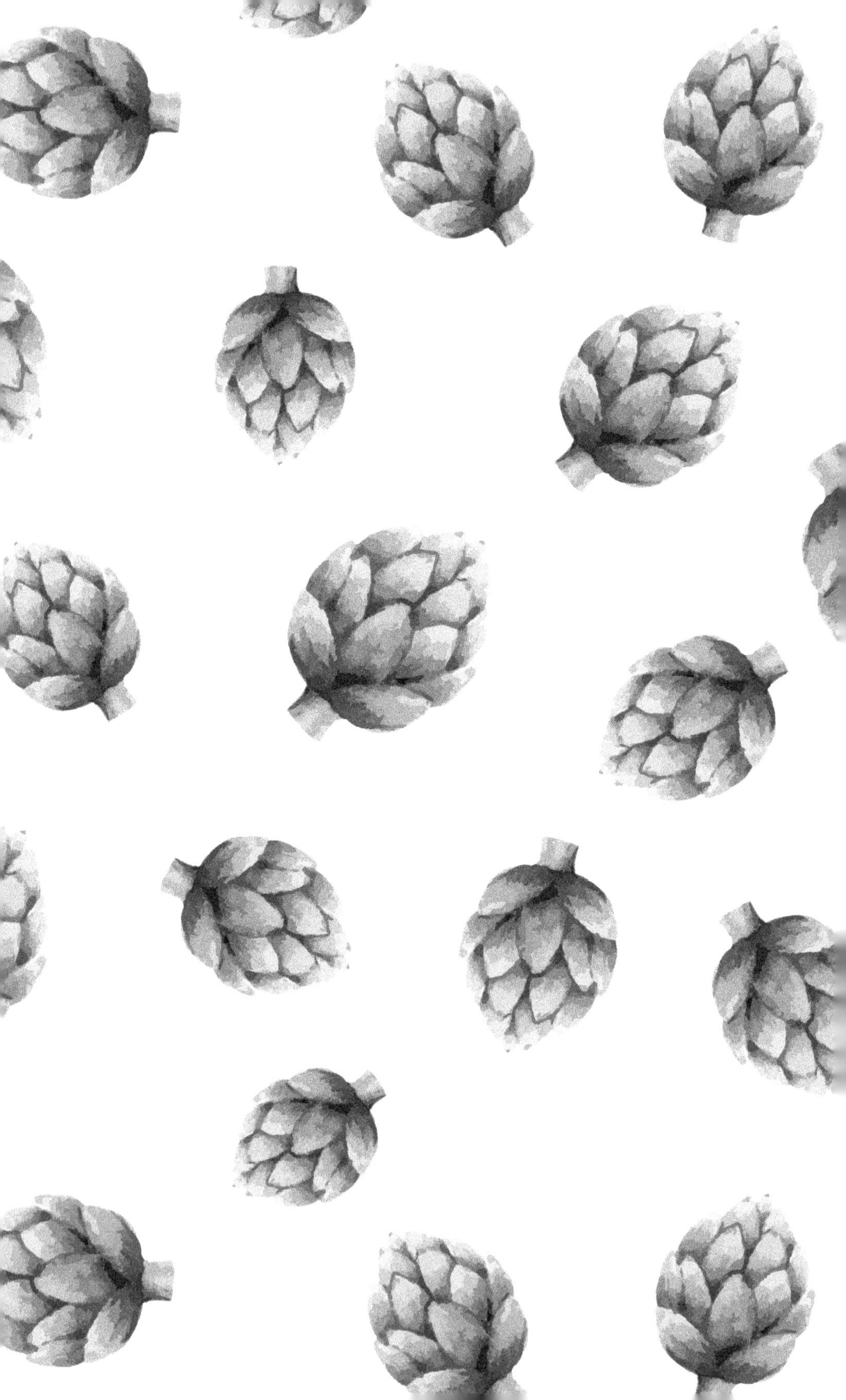

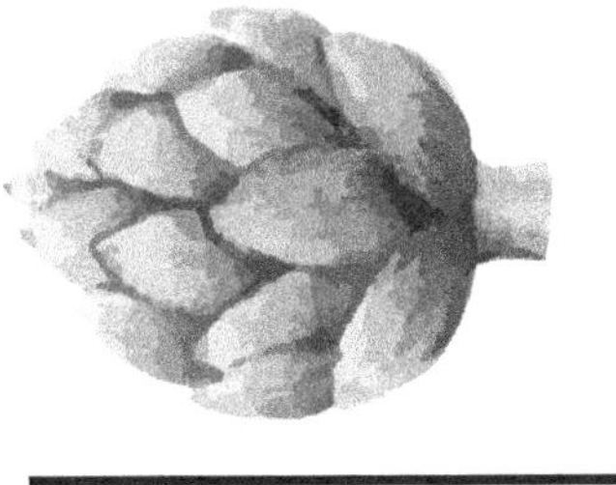
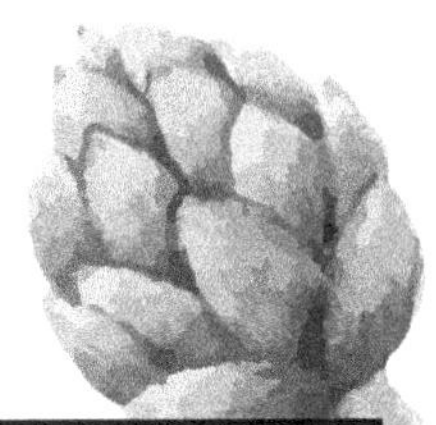
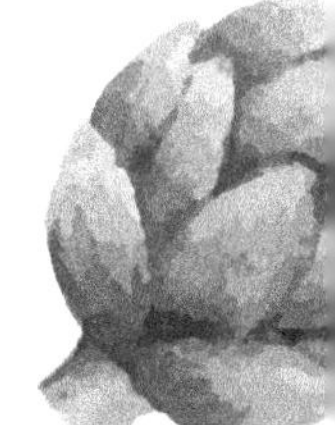

Savoury

Savoury treats make the perfect addition to a lunchbox as, most days, you are looking for a little more than just a salad. By adding something with a little more substance and a little more texture - a savoury snack offers that perfect bit of chew or crunch - it can make you feel totally satisfied.

By starting with salad as a base, the choice of my savoury addition is very seasonal. I tend to look for heavier, more filling options in the Winter or food that can easily be warmed up to help make you a little warmer.

All of these savoury options can be made ahead of time and stored in the fridge or freezer, making them easy to grab and throw in your lunchbox to save time when you need it.

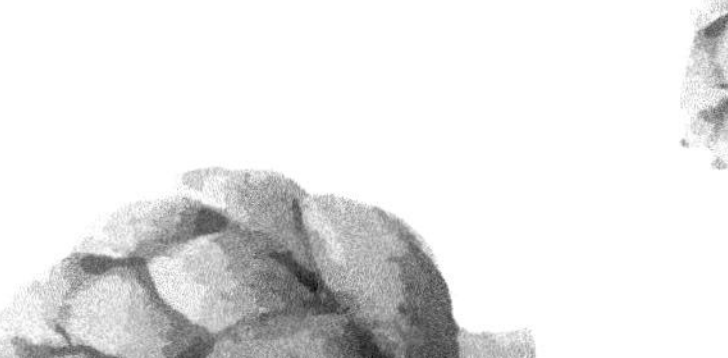
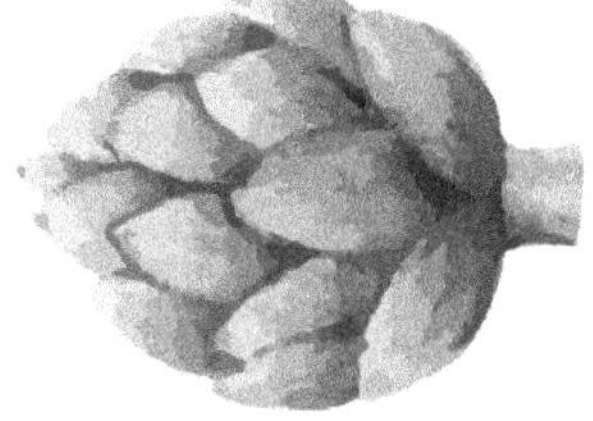
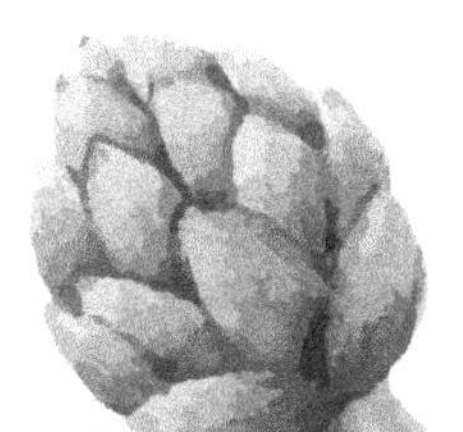

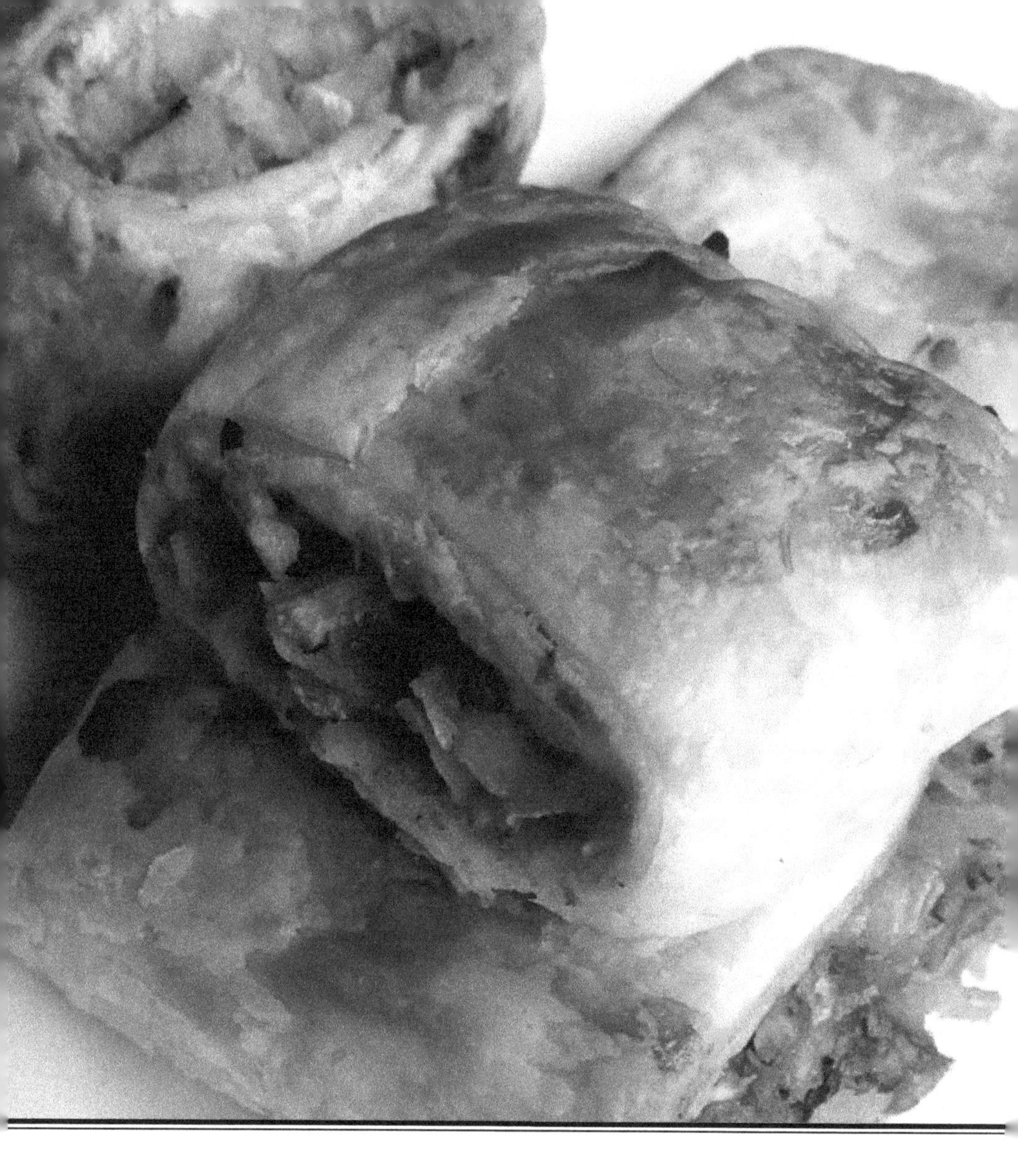

Veggie 'sausage' rolls

Whenever my brothers visit, my mum always bakes them her famous sausage rolls. She's been making these since we were little and as a child they were one of my favourite treats. Whenever I see and smell them, I can't help but reminisce and I really wanted to recreate that dish - but a version I could now enjoy. These vegetarian 'sausage' rolls are a great addition to any lunchbox, but they are especially great in the Winter as they're sure to warm you up and keep you full.

INGREDIENTS:

1 grated carrot
1 grated zucchini
1 small onion (finely diced)
2 medium grated potatoes
1 grated apple
125g crushed walnuts
1 egg
1 cup breadcrumbs
1/2 cup tomato relish
1/2 cup fresh parsley (chopped)

Sheets of puff pastry

METHOD:

Pre-heat the oven to 200 - 220 degrees Celsius.
Combine all the ingredients (except pastry).
Cut a sheet of puff pastry in half.
Spoon filling along the middle of the pastry.
Roll and cut into quarters.
Repeat until you have used all of the filling.
Brush with a little milk.
Bake for 12 - 15 minutes or until pastry is golden.

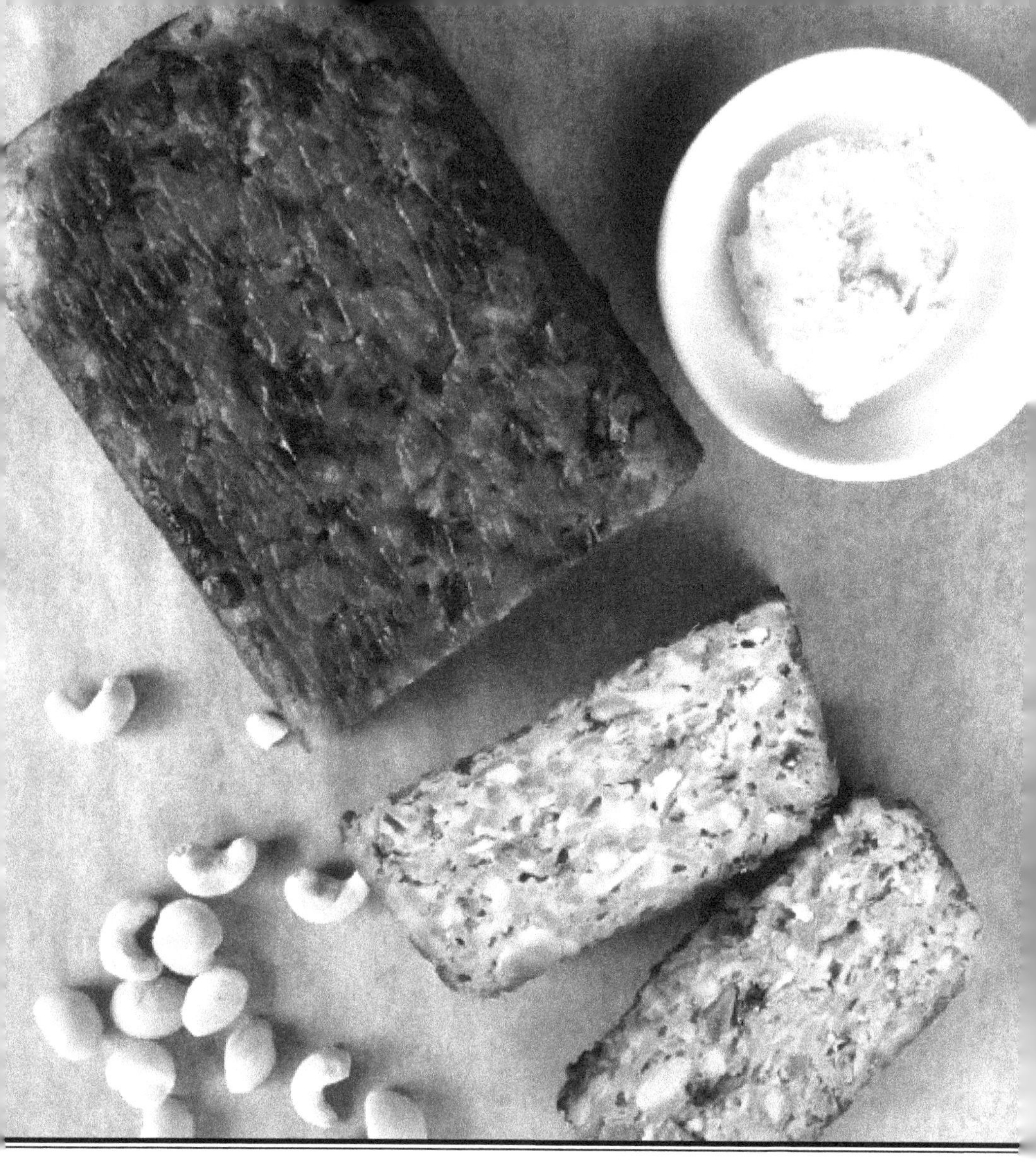

Nut loaf

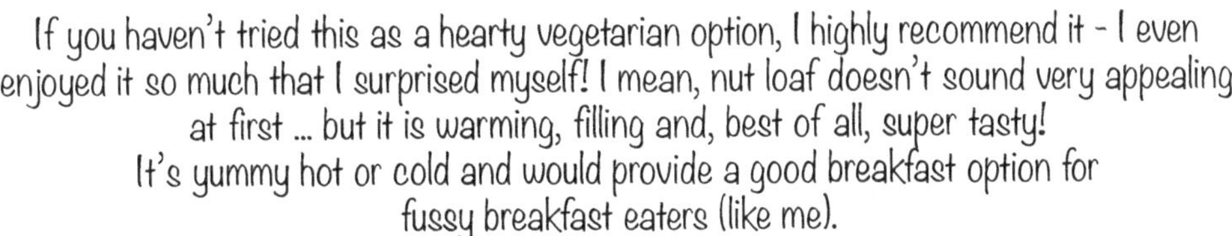

If you haven't tried this as a hearty vegetarian option, I highly recommend it - I even enjoyed it so much that I surprised myself! I mean, nut loaf doesn't sound very appealing at first ... but it is warming, filling and, best of all, super tasty!
It's yummy hot or cold and would provide a good breakfast option for fussy breakfast eaters (like me).

INGREDIENTS:

1/4 cup porcini mushrooms
200g nuts (I used cashews & macadamias)
2 slices of bread (I used light rye)
1 onion - chopped
4 celery stalks
2 field mushrooms
Olive oil
Clove of garlic
Chilli - finely diced
150g aborio rice
1/2 cup white wine
2 tablespoons light miso paste
500ml vegetable stock
1/2 cup grated cheese
2 eggs
Zest of 1 lemon
Handful chopped parsley

METHOD:

Soak porcini mushrooms in boiling water for 5 minutes.
Drain and discard liquid, chop and put aside.
Process nuts in food processor, put aside.
Pulse bread to create crumbs, put aside.

Sauté onion celery in olive oil for 5 mins or until soft.
Add garlic, chilli, and diced mushrooms, cook a further 2 minutes.
Add rice and cook for 2 minutes, then add white wine.
Stir through miso paste.
Meanwhile heat vegetable stock. Gradually add to rice mixture until absorbed (this will take around 20 mins).
Allow mixture to cool.
Add mushroom mixture, nuts, breadcrumbs, cheese, eggs, lemon zest and parsley to the cooked rice.
Spread into a loaf tin, cover in foil and cook for 45 minutes at 180 degrees Celsius.
Remove foil and cook a further 20 minutes or until golden on top.
Serve warm or cold. Store in fridge.

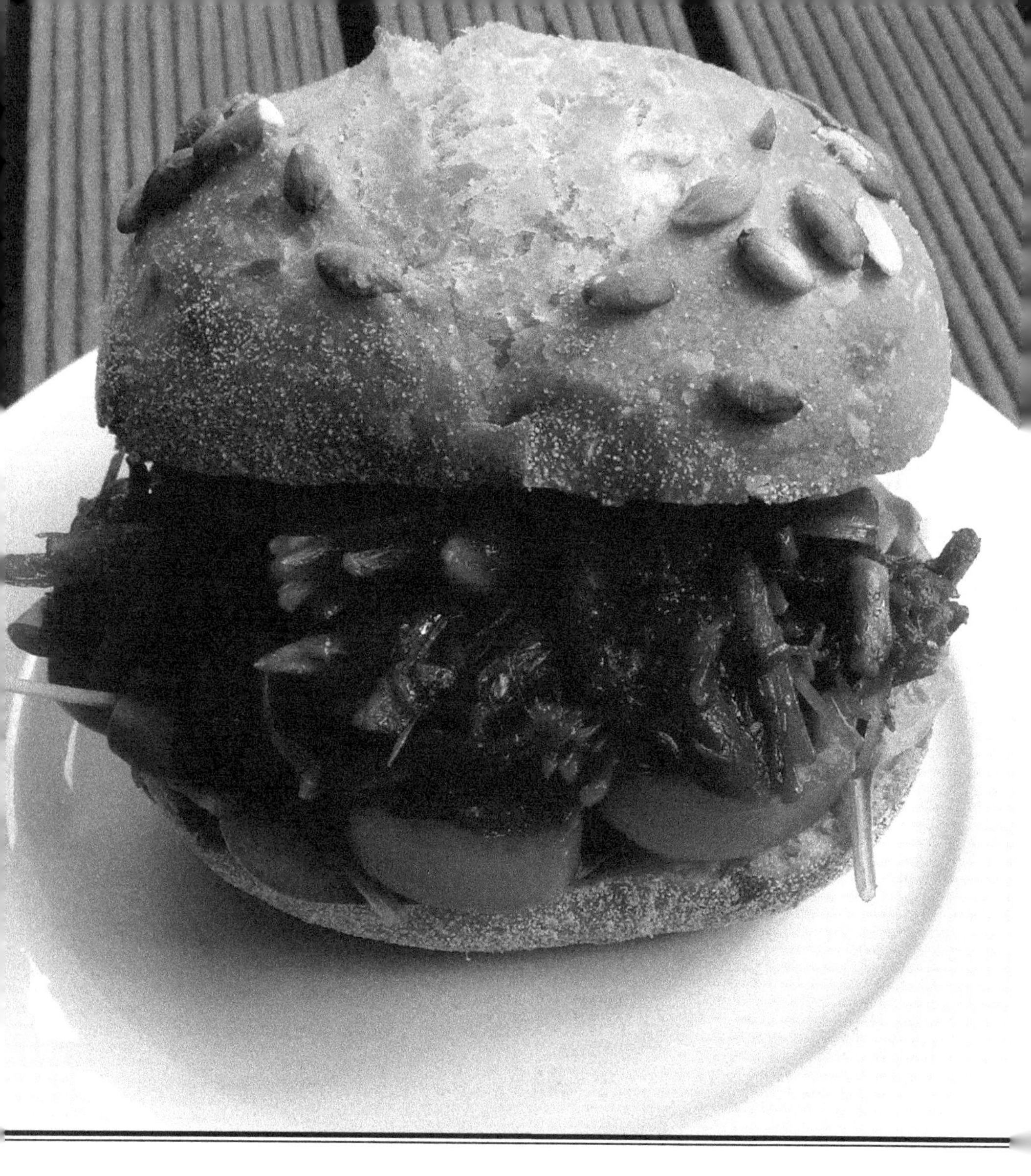

Pulled Jackfruit

A while ago I went out with friends in Melbourne and saw jackfruit tacos on the menu, but was too scared to try them. More recently I saw it again at a food truck. But as I approached the truck, it was rubbed off the board - sold out! However, I couldn't let the idea go! So after looking around town I finally found a can of jackfruit, in water (not syrup) at a local Asian grocer. The pulled jackfruit is actually quite easy to make and as the jackfruit itself has quite a neutral flavour, you can use different seasonings to get the taste you prefer.

INGREDIENTS:

1 540g can jackfruit in water
1 tablespoon brown sugar
1 teaspoon minced chilli
1/4 cup soy sauce
1 clove finely diced garlic
1 teaspoon Massal 'beef' stock powder
1/4 cup water
1 tablespoon coconut oil

METHOD:

Drain and rinse jackfruit.
Combine brown sugar, chilli, soy sauce, garlic, stock powder and 1/4 cup water in a bowl.
Cut the core pieces of the jackfruit away and discard.
Combine jackfruit with marinade.
Heat coconut oil in a large frypan.
Add jackfruit mixture and cook over a low temperature for up to 30 minutes.

Note - you will need to stir and check the fruit regularly, pulling it apart with 2 forks as it breaks down. You may also need to add additional water if required.

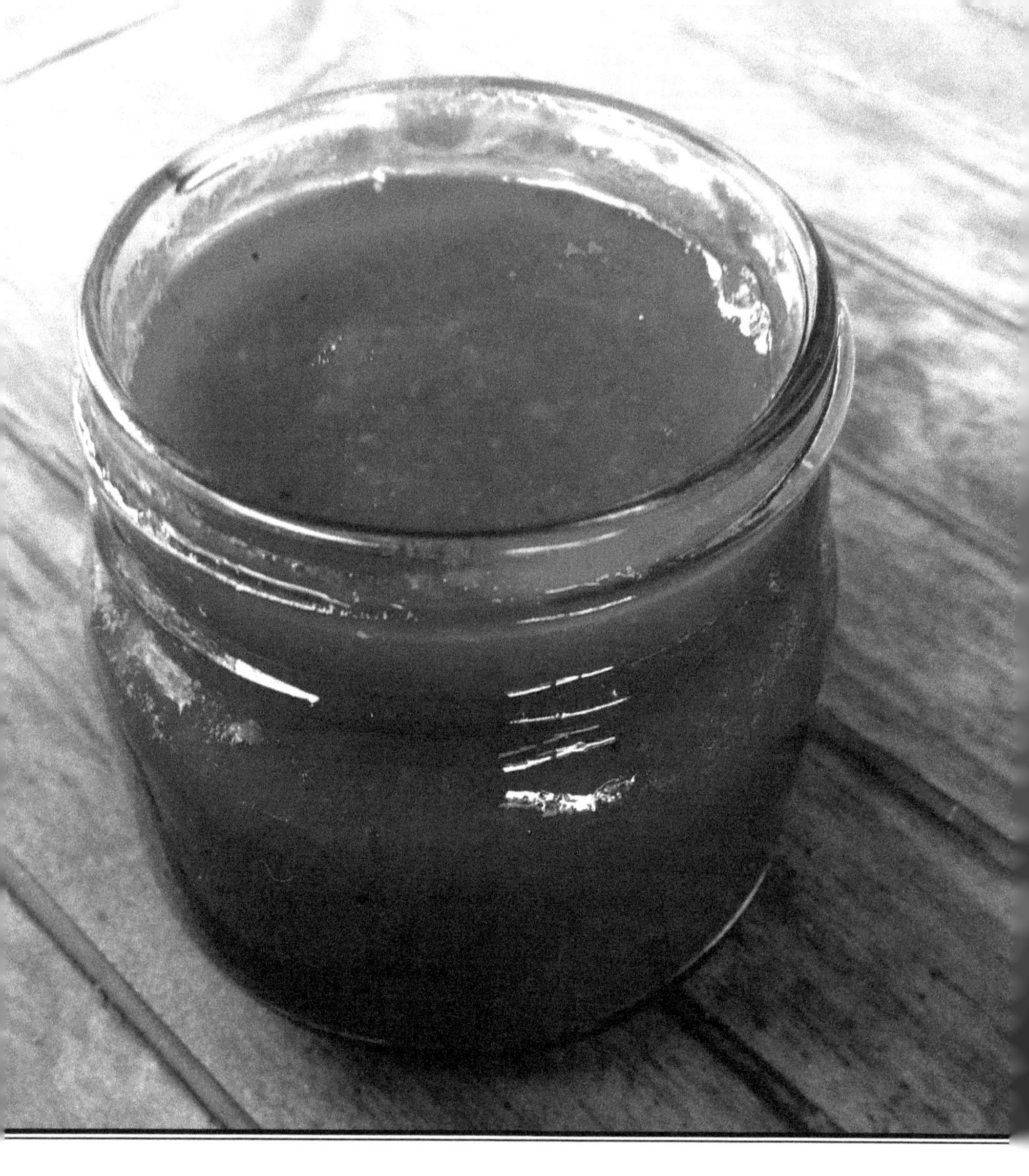

Beetroot soup

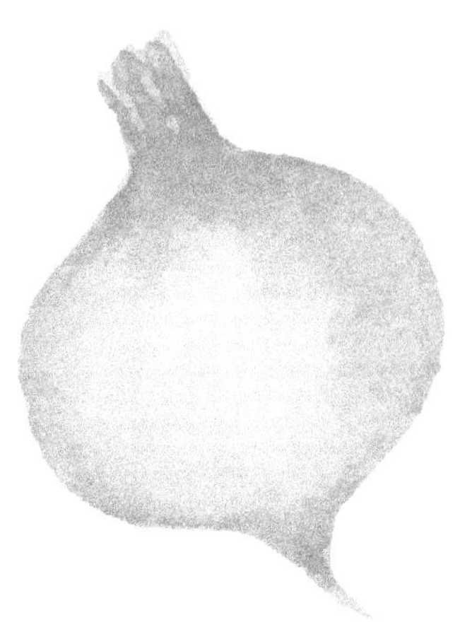

My favourite fresh juice combination is beetroot, apple and ginger - which is why I love this soup recipe so much. It combines those same ingredients, but with a savoury twist. One of the secrets when making this soup is to cook it low, covered and slow - so that the beetroot keeps that gorgeous deep purple colour. Sometimes I think my favourite colour is beetroot.

INGREDIENTS:

2 medium beetroot
1 Granny Smith apple
2 large carrots
1 onion
1 knob of ginger (grated)
Salt and pepper
5 cups vegetable stock

METHOD:

Peel and chop beetroot, apple, carrot, ginger and onion into small pieces. Place in a roasting tray.
Cover with the 5 cups of vegetable stock.
Season with salt and pepper.
Cover with foil and cook at 140 degrees Celsius for 4 hours.
Allow to cool slightly, then puree.

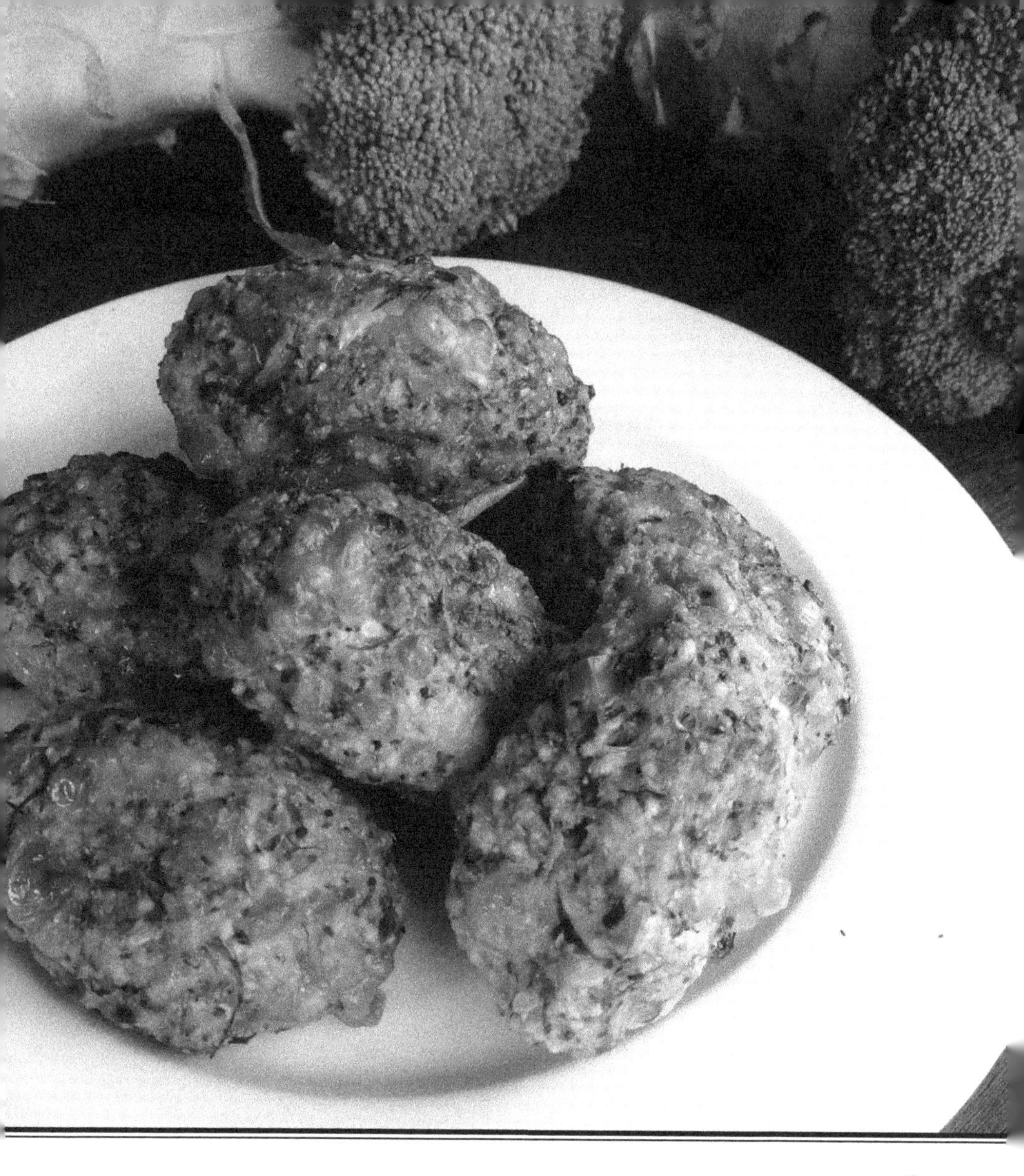

Broccoli nuggets

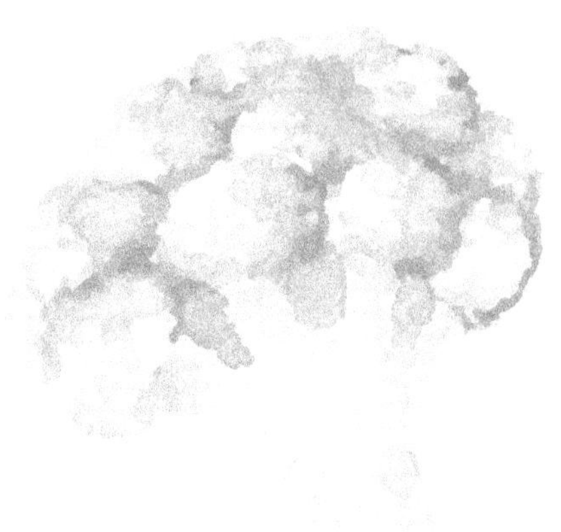

When you are packing lunches for boys (or girls) on the go, snacks they can eat with their hands make them happy. Snacks that are full of veggies make ME happy. Broccoli nuggets are perfect, they are moreish and so easy to make. I am honestly going to have to start doubling the recipe. By the time they have cooled on the tray ready to go into the fridge for lunches, half have usually disappeared!

INGREDIENTS:

1 head of broccoli
1 slice of bread
1/2 cup grated tasty cheese
1/2 an onion (finely diced)
2 spring onions, chopped
1/2 cup panko bread crumbs
2 eggs
1/2 cup fresh herbs, chopped (e.g. parsley and dill)

METHOD:

Preheat oven to 180 degrees Celsius.
Cut broccoli into florets. Remove outer part of the stem and cut the rest into small pieces.
Process florets and stem to create broccoli crumbs.
Remove broccoli crumbs and transfer to a bowl.
Process bread and combine with broccoli crumbs.
Add cheese, finely diced onion, chopped spring onions, panko bread crumbs, eggs and chopped herbs and mix until combined.
Take a spoonful of the mixture and squeeze between your hands - the mixture will naturally take shape.
Place on a tray lined with baking paper and bake for 25 - 30 minutes.

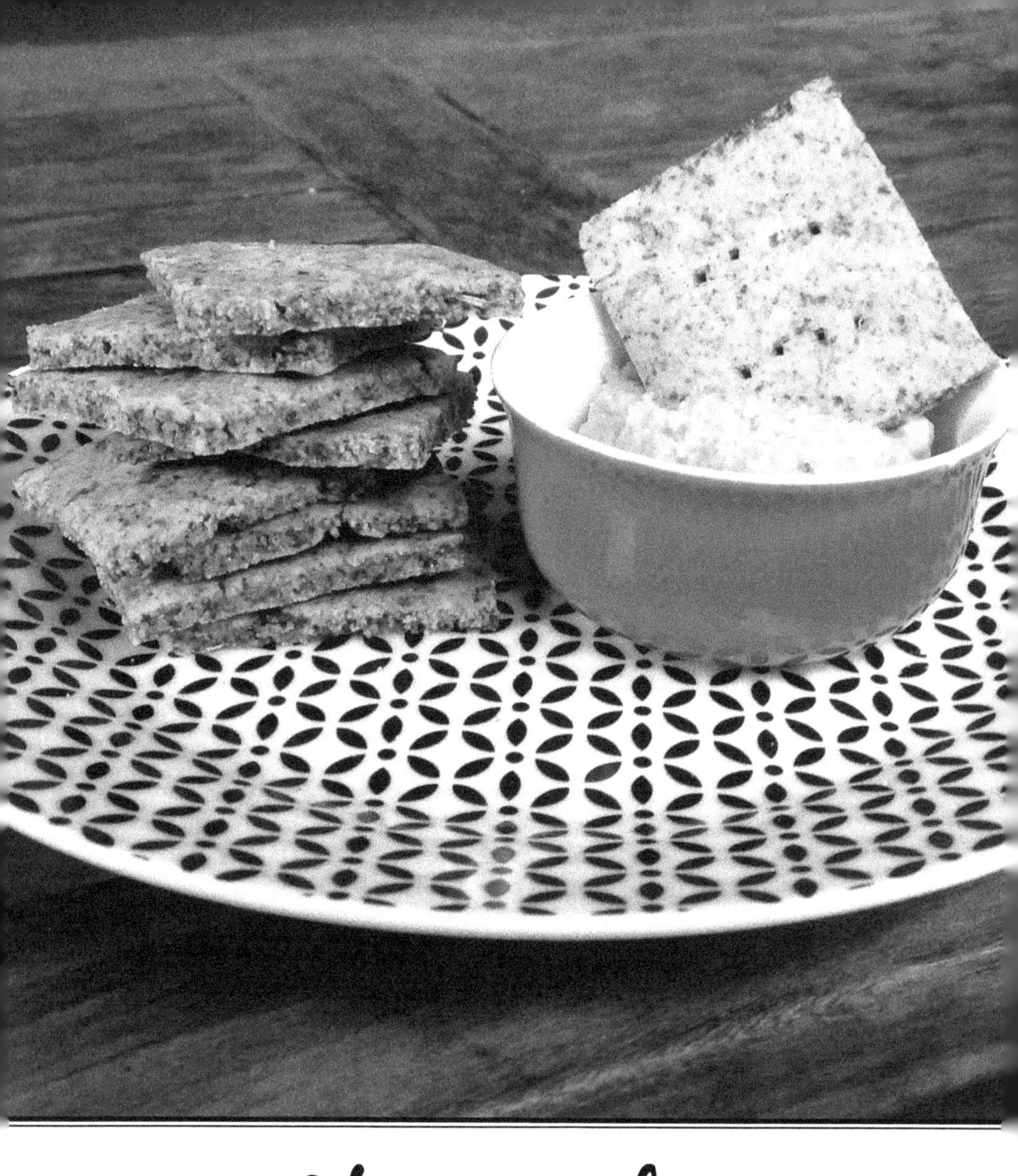

Herby chickpea crackers

My weekly baking projects often celebrate sweet treats. However this recipe for Herby Chickpea Crackers is a great example of a home-cooked savoury snack. If you've never had a go at baking your own biscuits it is well worth a try, and easier than you may think. You can easily change the flavour by using a different flavoured salt or by experimenting with the dried herbs.

INGREDIENTS:

1 cup chickpea (besan) flour
2 tablespoons LSA
Pinch of baking soda
1 tablespoons olive oil
1/2 teaspoon garlic salt
1/4 cup water
2 tablespoons mixed dry herbs and/or dried rosemary

METHOD:

Combine all ingredients to create a dough.
Roll out the dough between 2 sheets of baking paper, as thin as possible.
Remove top layer of paper.
Cut into squares and prick each square with a fork.
Bake at 180 degrees Celsius for 20 minutes.
Allow to cool, then gently break apart.

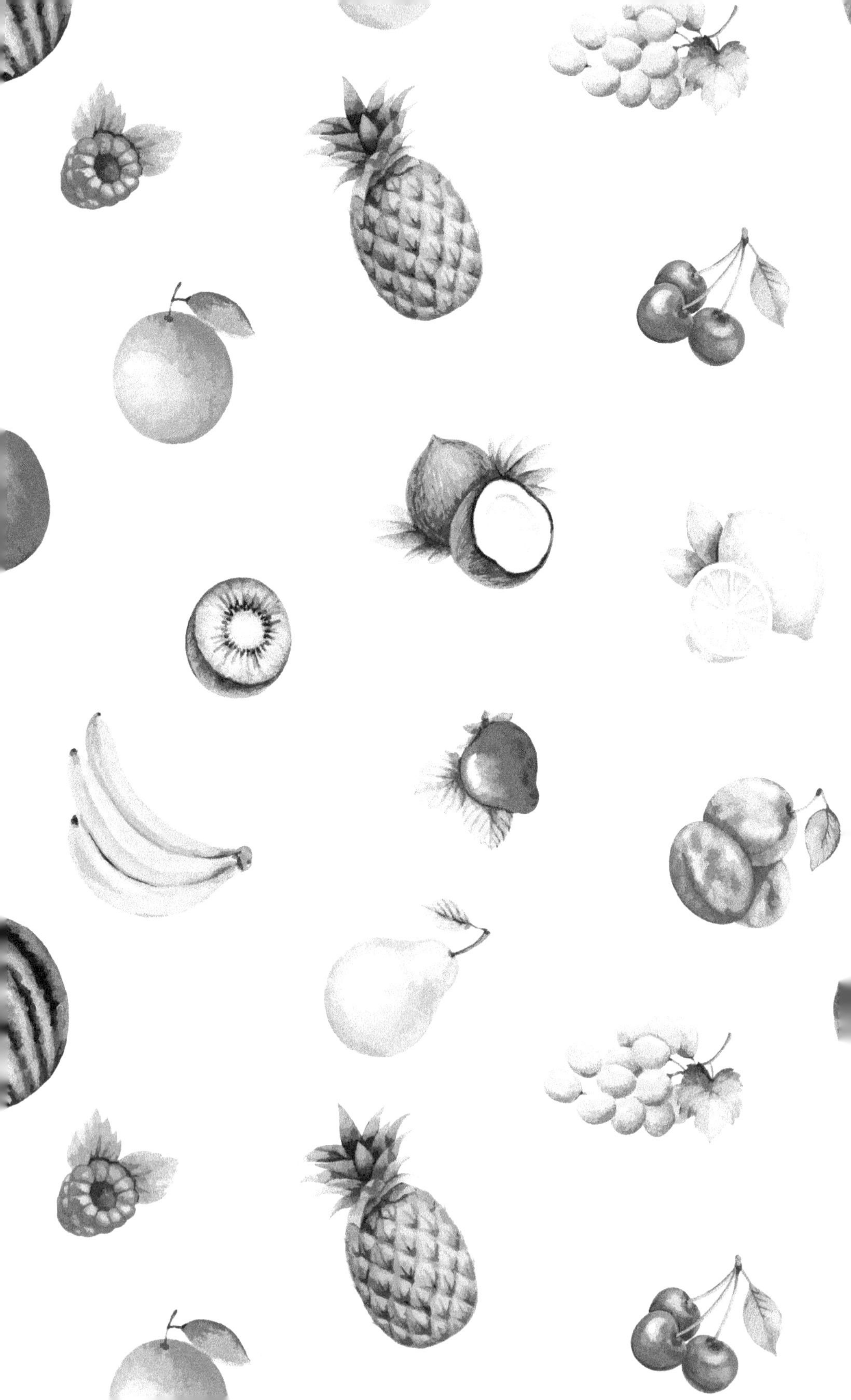

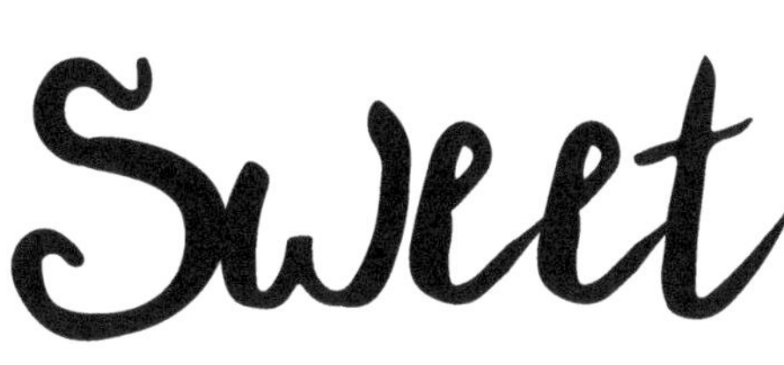

And now for everyone's favourite part...the sweet treats! Whilst these are made using healthier options and are not filled with loads of preservatives or refined sugars, they are still meant to be treats and therefore eaten in moderation.

I usually add one sweet treat to my lunchbox, along with one or two pieces of fruit. This gives a lovely finish to lunch and makes you feel as though you have eaten a full and proper meal - even when you're on the run!

All of these options can be made ahead of time and it is a great idea to have some ready to go in your freezer so that you're not caught out craving something sweet and then making an unhealthy choice.

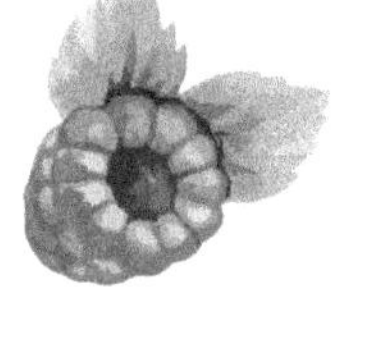

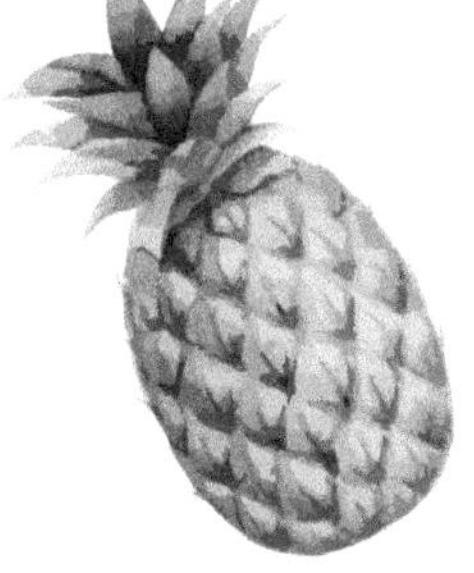

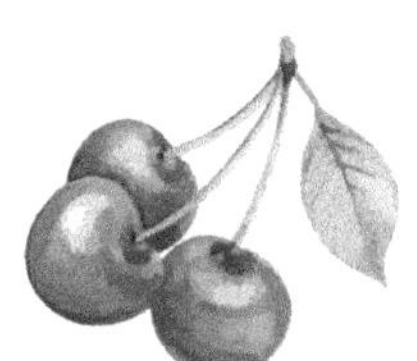

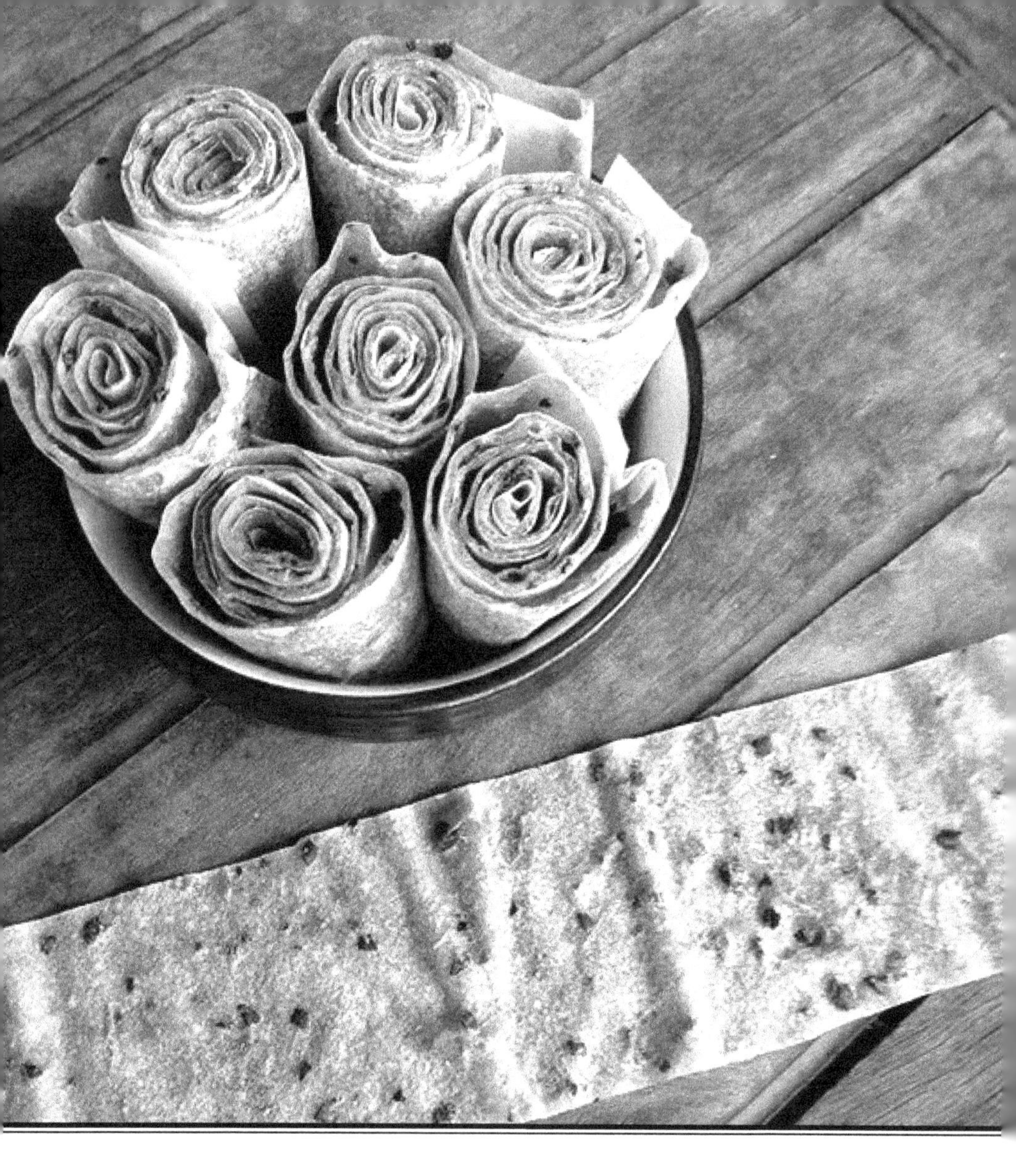

Fruit Leather

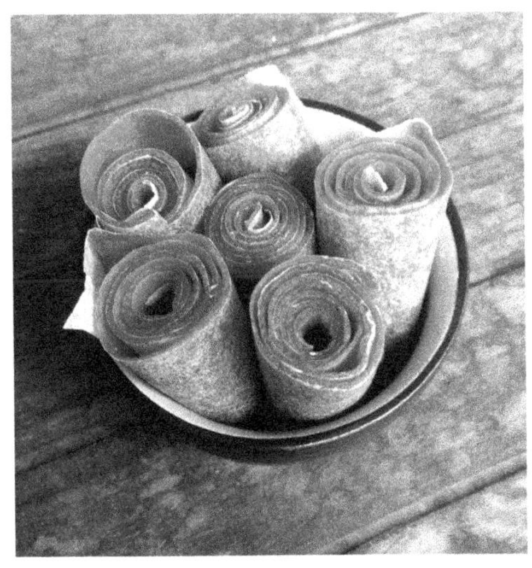

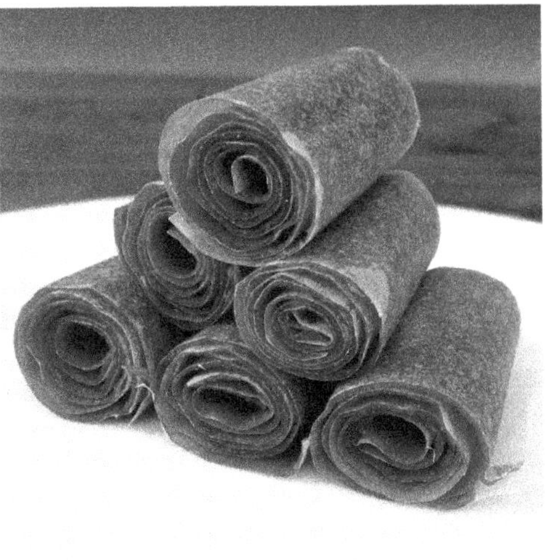

This is a great way to use up excess fruit over Summer. Even if the fruit is a little bruised or old - it can still be turned into a beautiful snack using this recipe. I've got three different versions here (apple, pineapple & passionfruit - shown left, peach & nectarine or apricot - shown above) but I encourage you to experiment and have fun with whatever fruit you enjoy!

INGREDIENTS:

Peach & Nectarine
3 cups of chopped peaches and nectarines
Juice of 1 lemon

Apricot
3 cups chopped apricots
Juice of 1 lemon

Apple, Pineapple & Passionfruit
6 small Granny Smith apples (or 3 normal ones)
1 1/2 cups chopped pineapple
Pulp of 5 passionfruit
Juice of 1 lemon

METHOD:

Halve and remove stones from the fruit.
Place all ingredients in a medium saucepan and cook over a low heat for 20 - 30 minutes.
After this time the liquid will leave the fruit and it will begin breaking down.
Remove from heat and allow to cool for 10 minutes.
Blend mixture until smooth.
Line a large baking tray with 2 sheets of baking paper.
Spread the mixture over the baking paper. Make sure it is quite thin and even.
Set the oven to the lowest possible temperature (around 100 degrees Celsius) and leave for at least 5 hours or even overnight.
The mixture should be completely dry - if there are still damp spots, return to the oven for a little longer.
Once completely dry, remove from the oven and allow to cool.
Leaving one sheet of baking paper attached, cut the mixture into strips and roll up.

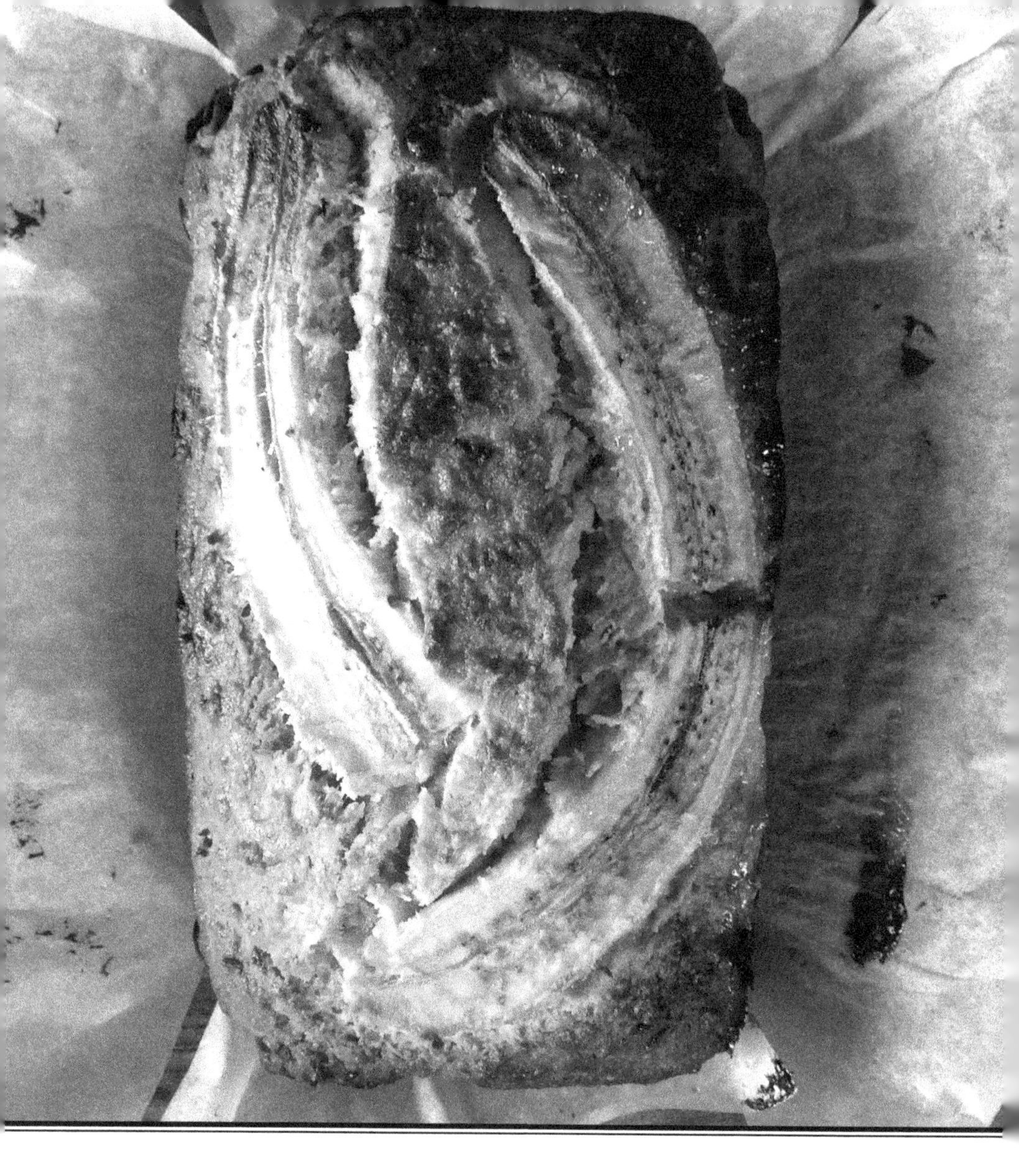

Banana bread

I love it when we have over-ripe bananas, especially if they are going black and squishy. Why? Because this banana bread recipe is amazing. It is super easy to make. It will keep for several days in an airtight container or can be sliced and frozen, wrapped in baking paper. It makes a nutritious breakfast, just pop the wrapped slice straight into a sandwich press to thaw and toast. It is a filling lunch box snack and it is absolutely lovely toasted with a dollop of coconut yogurt.

INGREDIENTS:

Dry
1 1/2 cups spelt flour
1/2 teaspoon bicarbonate soda
1 teaspoon baking powder
1 cup desiccated coconut
1/4 cup coconut sugar

Wet
4 ripe bananas, mashed
2 eggs
2/3 cup coconut oil (melted)
1/4 cup maple syrup

METHOD:

Preheat oven to 180 Celsius.
Combine dry ingredients in a bowl.
Mash bananas, stir in other wet ingredients and stir until combined.
Make a well in dry ingredients. Stir through wet ingredients and mix until completely combined.
Pour mixture into lightly greased loaf tin lined with baking paper.
Place fresh fruit on top of loaf (optional - but I've used banana here, and I also love it with fresh figs baked into the top!)
Bake for 45 minutes.

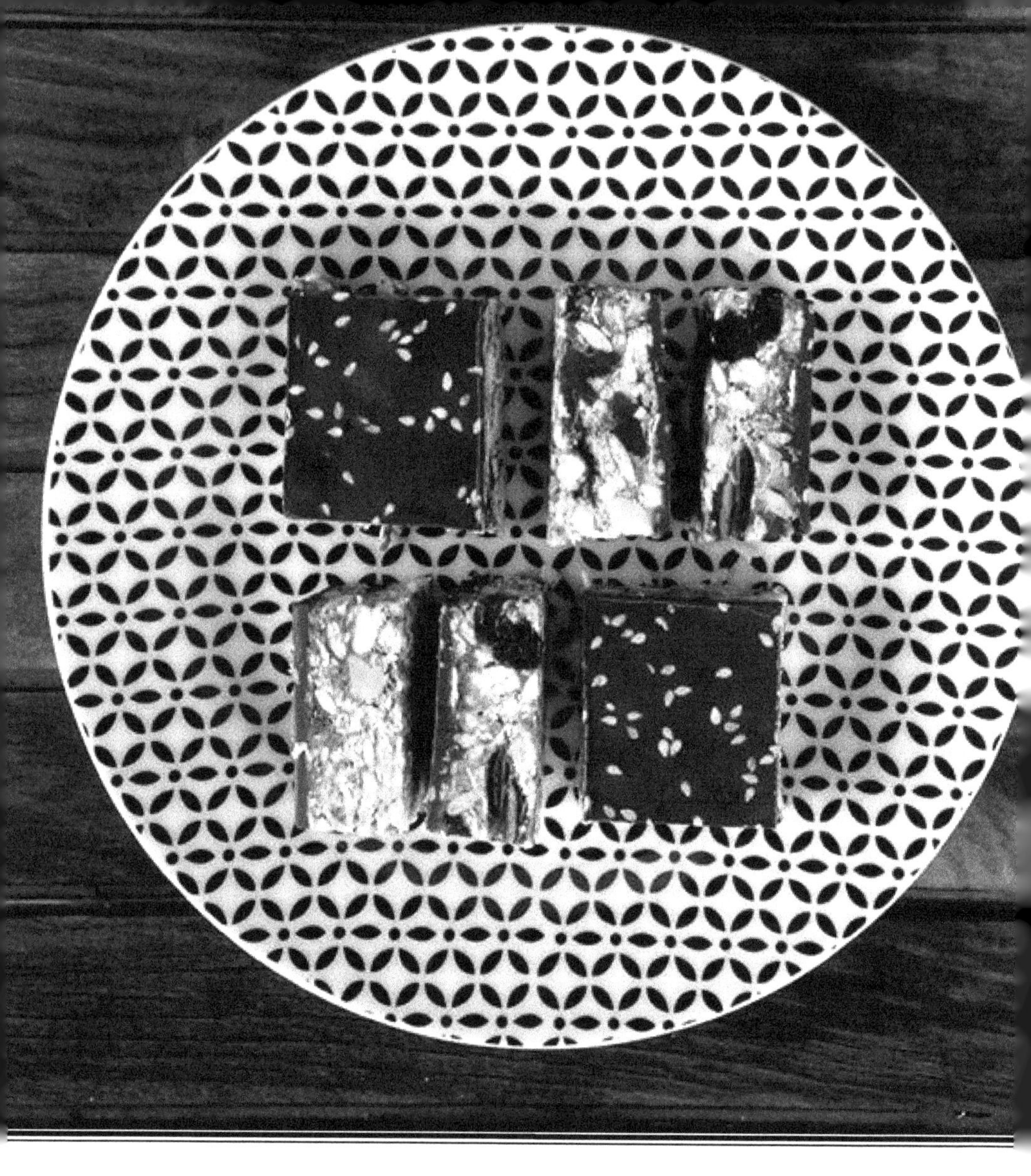

1 + 1 + 1 slice

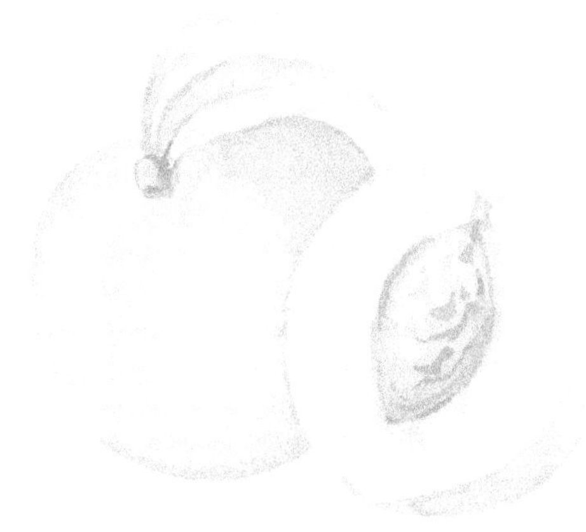

This is my husband's favourite slice. I love it because of the simple '1 cup of nuts + 1 cup of seeds + 1 cup of dried fruit' formula - it means I can use whatever's in my pantry to finish off all those packets that just have a little bit of this or a little bit of that leftover. However, I usually work with combinations of two: 2 Types of seeds, 2 types of nut and 2 types of fruit - but it is so easy to adapt and use whatever you have on hand.

INGREDIENTS:

Decide on your 1 + 1 + 1:
1 cup of seeds (eg. chia, sunflower, sesame, hemp or pumpkin seeds),
1 cup of nuts (eg. macadamias, cashews, almonds walnuts or pistachios),
1 cup dried fruit (eg. dried apricots, dried cranberries, dates, dried pineapple)

1 cup of rolled oats
1/2 cup desiccated coconut
1/2 cup honey
1/4 cup maple syrup
1/2 cup tahini
1/2 cup flaxseed meal
2 tablespoons coconut oil
A block of good quality, fair trade chocolate

METHOD:

Place seeds, nuts and fruit on an oven tray lined with baking paper along with oats and desiccated coconut.
Put honey, maple syrup and tahini in ramekins and place on the tray.
Put the tray in the oven for 30 mins at 100 degrees Celsius.
Place warm ingredients in a bowl and add flaxseed meal. Mix until combined.
Press into a tin and place in the fridge.
Melt chocolate and coconut oil and pour over the top.
Sprinkle with sesame seeds.

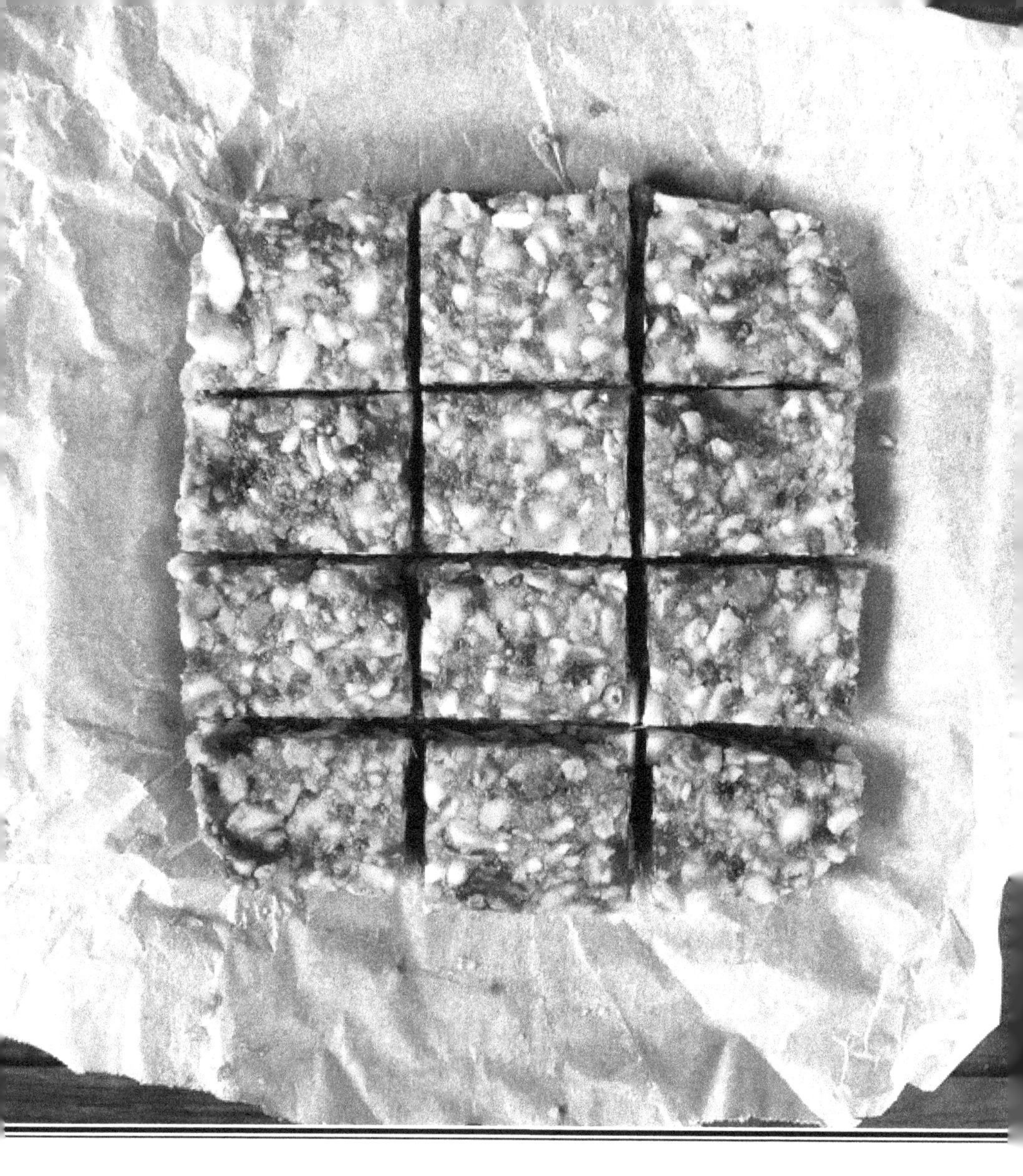

Bek's date & nut slice

My sister-in-law took a slice, similar to this one, away on a family camping trip. Once I'd tried it I was keen to make it myself. Firstly, because it was delicious but also as it has so few ingredients and is easy to make. In Bek's version, she used shredded coconut, but when I made it I replaced that with sunflower seeds. The beauty of this recipe is you can easily adapt it to suit your own tastes, or to accommodate whatever you happen to have in the pantry.

INGREDIENTS:

1 cup of nuts (I've used 1/2 cup cashews & 1/2 cup almonds)
12 medjool dates
1/4 cup sunflower seeds
1 1/2 tablespoons coconut oil

METHOD:

Briefly process nuts, you want to keep some chunks in the mixture.
Remove nuts from processor .
Process the medjool dates and coconut oil until a smooth paste forms.
Combine nuts, seeds and date mixture and press into a tray.
Store in the fridge.

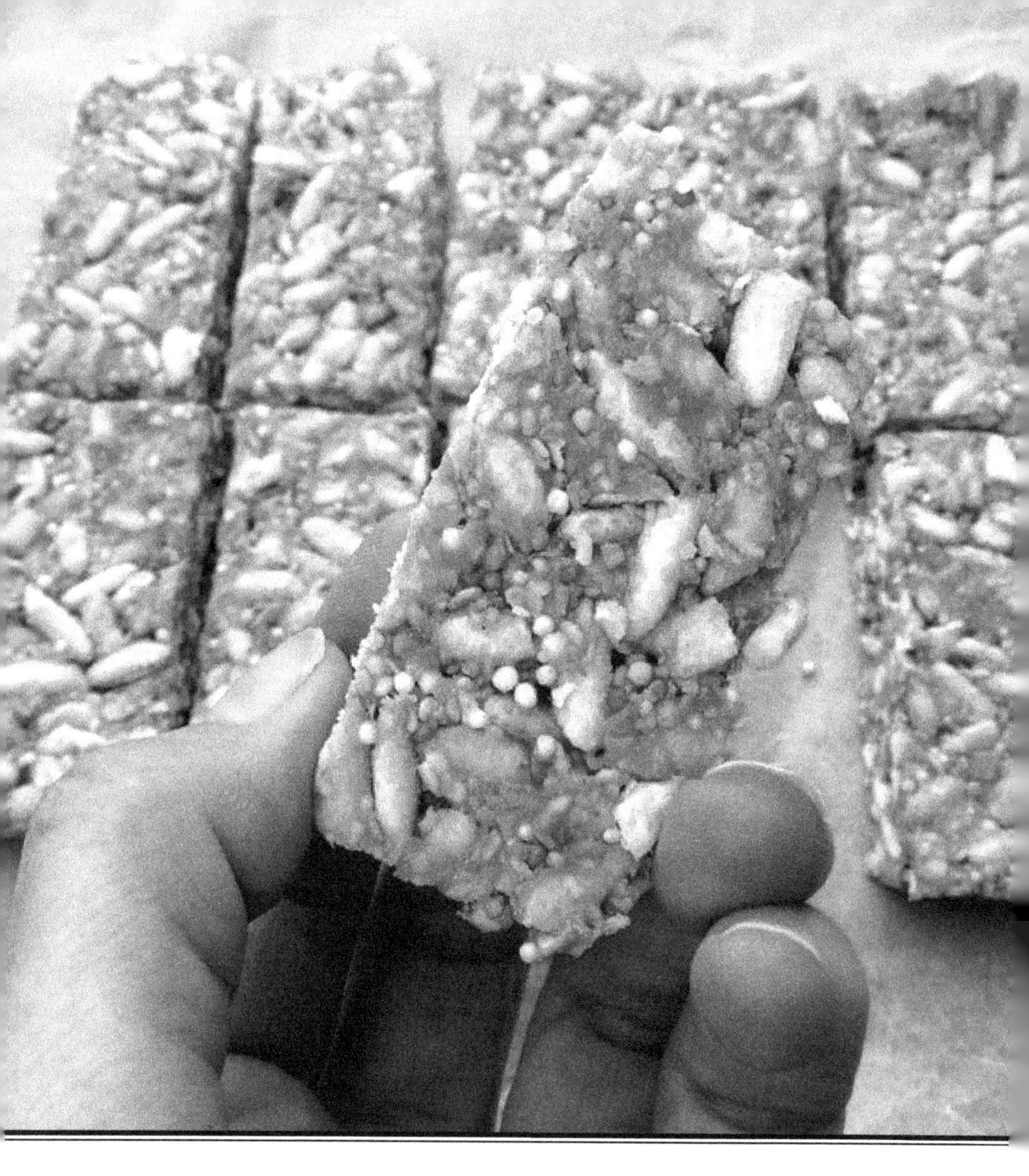

Funfetti slice

The only time I have supplemented my diet with protein powder was when I was long distance running. When I was left with some after an event, I would use it to make this protein rich slice. In my version, I have used Inca Inchi powder, however you could use whatever protein powder you may have. I love Inca Inchi powder as it is made from nuts rather than chemical or whey protein so it is suitable for vegans and it has a lovely nutty flavour.

INGREDIENTS:

1/2 cup oats
3 tablespoons Inca Inchi or Protein Powder
1 cup puffed brown rice
1/4 teaspoon sea salt
3 tablespoons natural peanut butter
5 tablespoons honey
1 teaspoon vanilla paste
Naturally coloured sprinkles

METHOD:

Process oats until they are a powder like consistency.
Combine in a bowl with the Inca Inchi powder, puffed rice, sprinkles and sea salt.
Meanwhile, gently heat the peanut butter, honey and vanilla over a low heat until combined.
Pour over dry ingredients. Mix until combined and press into a square tin.
Add additional sprinkles to the top of the slice.
Set in the fridge then cut into bars.

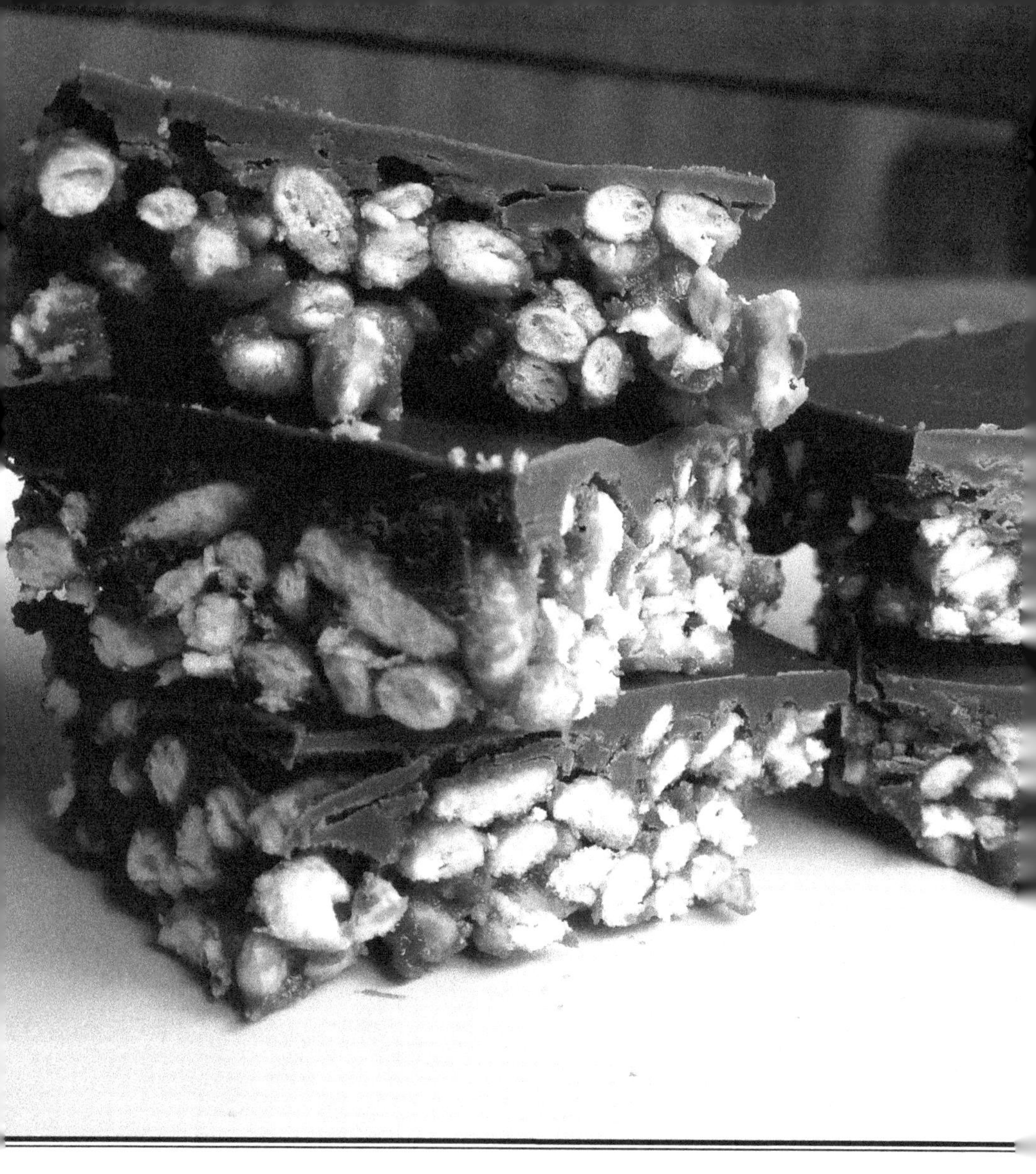

Choc-rice slice

The first time I made this slice, I didn't write the recipe down – I was just happily adding ingredients I had in the pantry that I wanted to use up. But the family enjoyed it, so I had to retrace my steps to recall and record a recipe. When my husband or the boys cook something new, they always stick to the recipe, and measure everything accurately. I remember my eldest watching me cook one day and commenting, "you are so ... approximate!" This is something I've definitely had to work on to create and share content on Instagram. Recipes such as this one have journeyed from 'kitchen experiment' to 'tried and tested.'

INGREDIENTS:

½ cup cacao peanut spread (or your favourite peanut butter and a tablespoon of cacao)
½ cup rice malt syrup
1 teaspoon vanilla paste
Pinch Himalayan salt
4 cups puffed brown rice
120g good quality, fair trade, dark chocolate or vegan chocolate.

METHOD:

Combine peanut butter, rice malt syrup vanilla and salt over low heat until combined.
Stir through 4 cups puffed brown rice.
Press into tin lined with baking paper and allow to set in the fridge.
Meanwhile melt chocolate of your choice.
Pour over the top of the slice and return to the fridge.

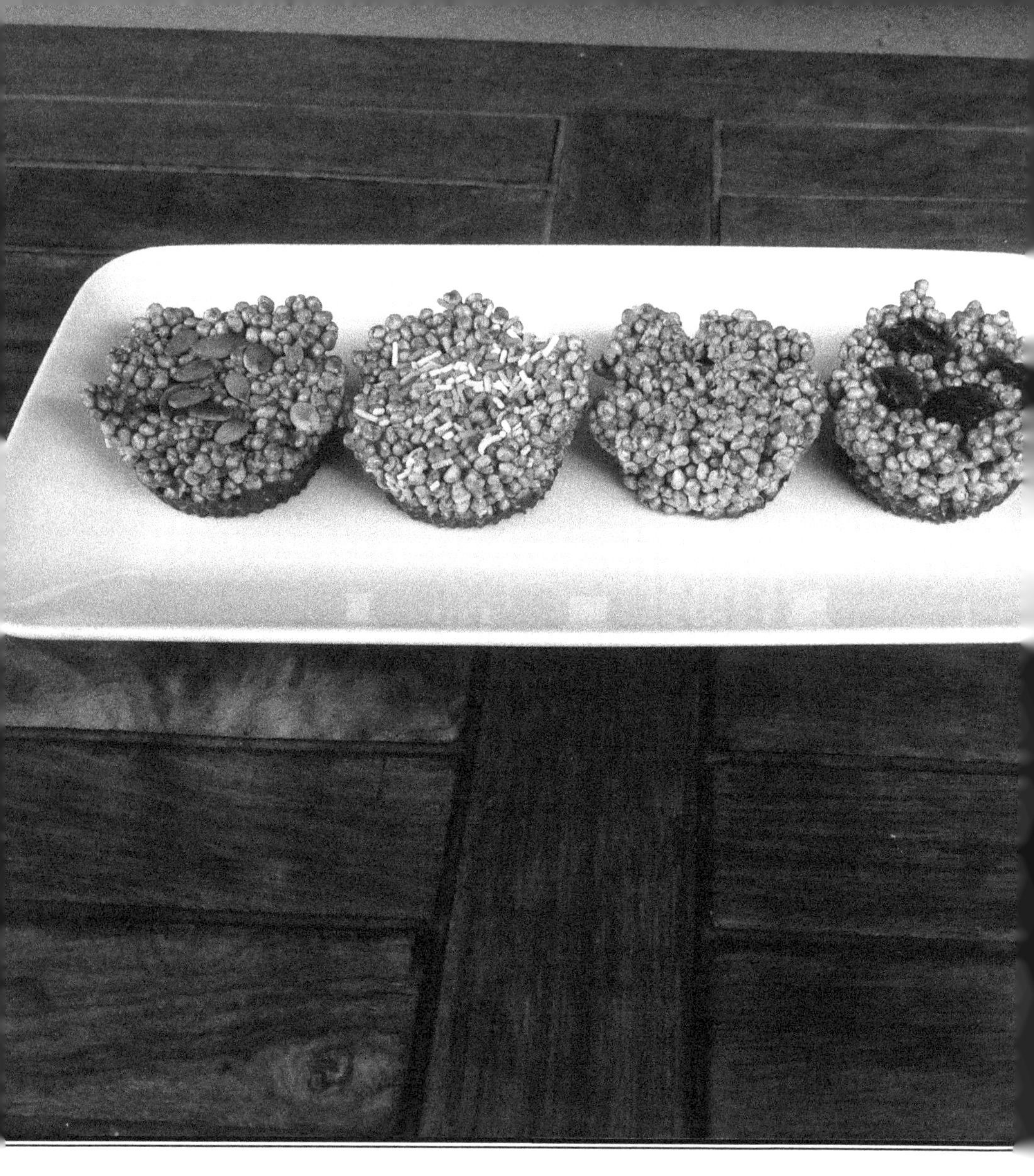

Chocolate crackles

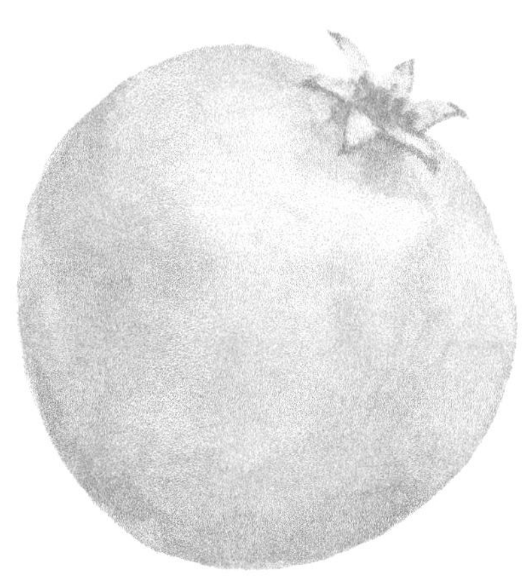

Remember chocolate crackles? They were one of the ultimate party food treats when I was a kid! My goal with this recipe was to create a healthier alternative. In this version I've used puffed millet in place of the usual popular breakfast cereal. Puffed brown rice is another alternative. When it comes to 'sprinkles' you can be as creative as you like. On different occasions I've used ingredients like: cranberries, hemp seeds, pumpkin seeds, buckinis or even naturally coloured sprinkles. They all add colour and a little bit of fun.

INGREDIENTS:

1/3 cup coconut oil
1/4 cup cacao
1/4 cup honey
2 cups puffed millet

Optional:
Pumpkin seeds
Hemp seeds
1/2 cup dried cranberries
Buckinis
Sprinkles

METHOD:

Heat coconut oil, cacao and honey over a low heat until melted and combined.
Stir through puffed millet.
Share between silicone mould (small or large).
Sprinkle with optional extras.
Place in fridge until set.

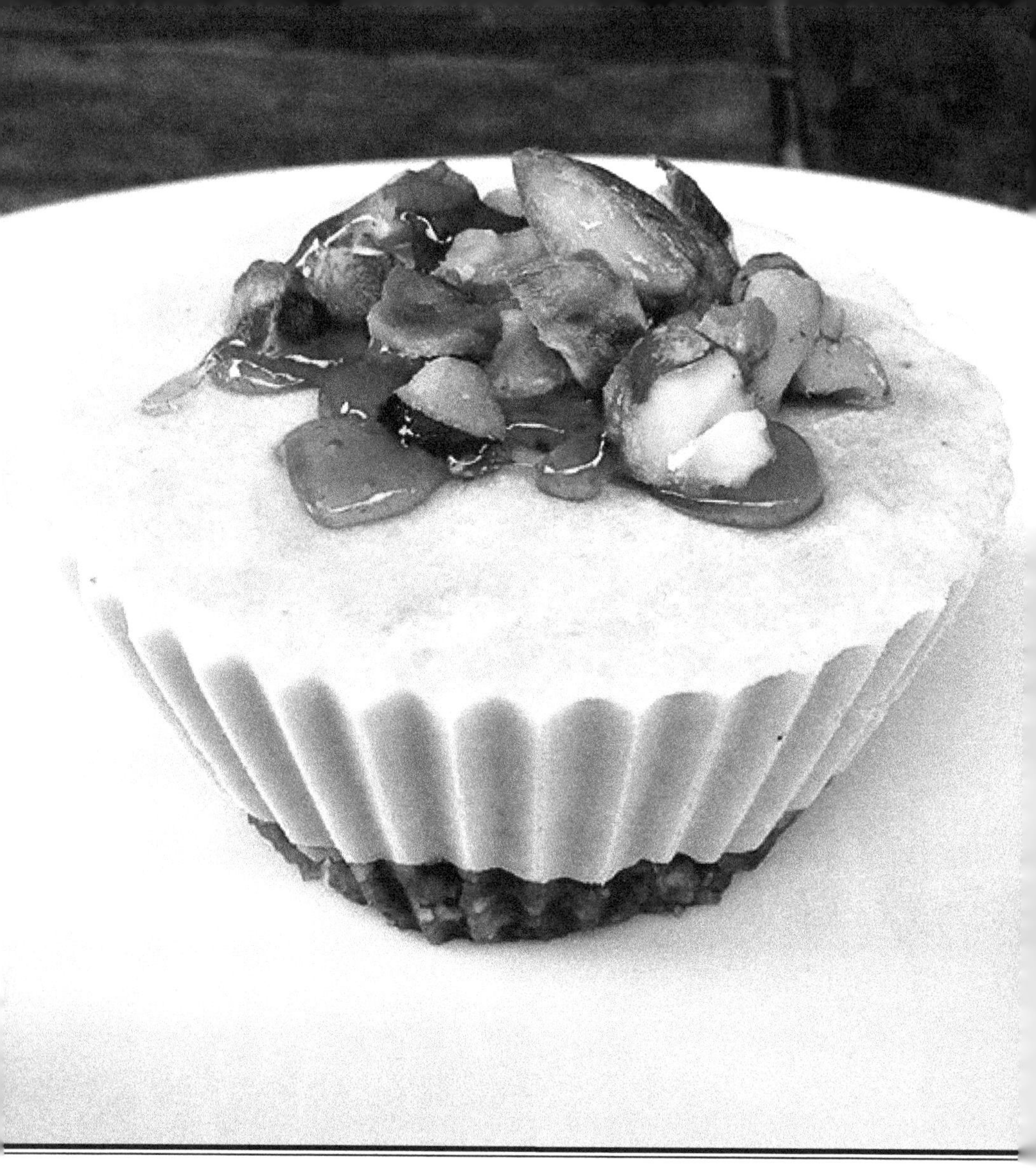

Raw fig cheesecake

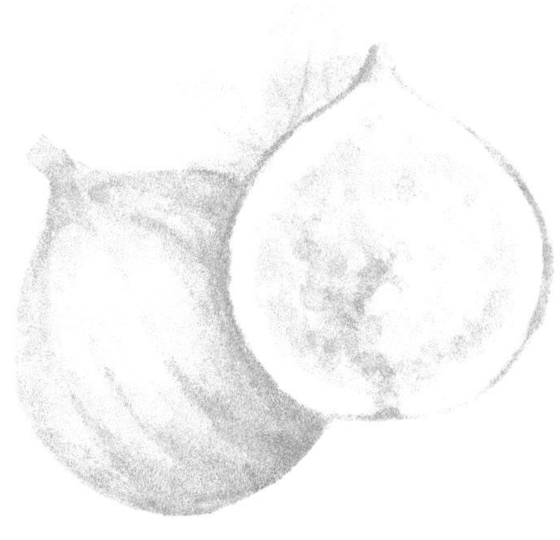

You don't need to turn on the oven to enjoy cake. This dessert is raw, vegan and includes wholesome ingredients. You will be surprised at just how creamy and delicious this vegan take on 'cheesecake' is - thanks to the inclusion of both cashews and coconut cream. If figs are not available, try substituting berries for another tasty raw treat.

INGREDIENTS:

Base
10 medjool dates
150g blanched almonds
1/2 cup desiccated coconut
1 tablespoon coconut oil (melted)
Pinch of pink Himalayan rock salt

Filling
2 cups soaked cashews
400 ml coconut cream
1 teaspoon vanilla paste
6 fresh figs
1/4 cup coconut syrup

METHOD:

Process ingredients for base until well combined.
Press into one large tin or 12 muffin size silicone moulds.

Blend filling ingredients until combined, pour over base(s) and place in the freezer until set.

Note: to soak cashews, cover with water for 4 hours.
Drain water before use.

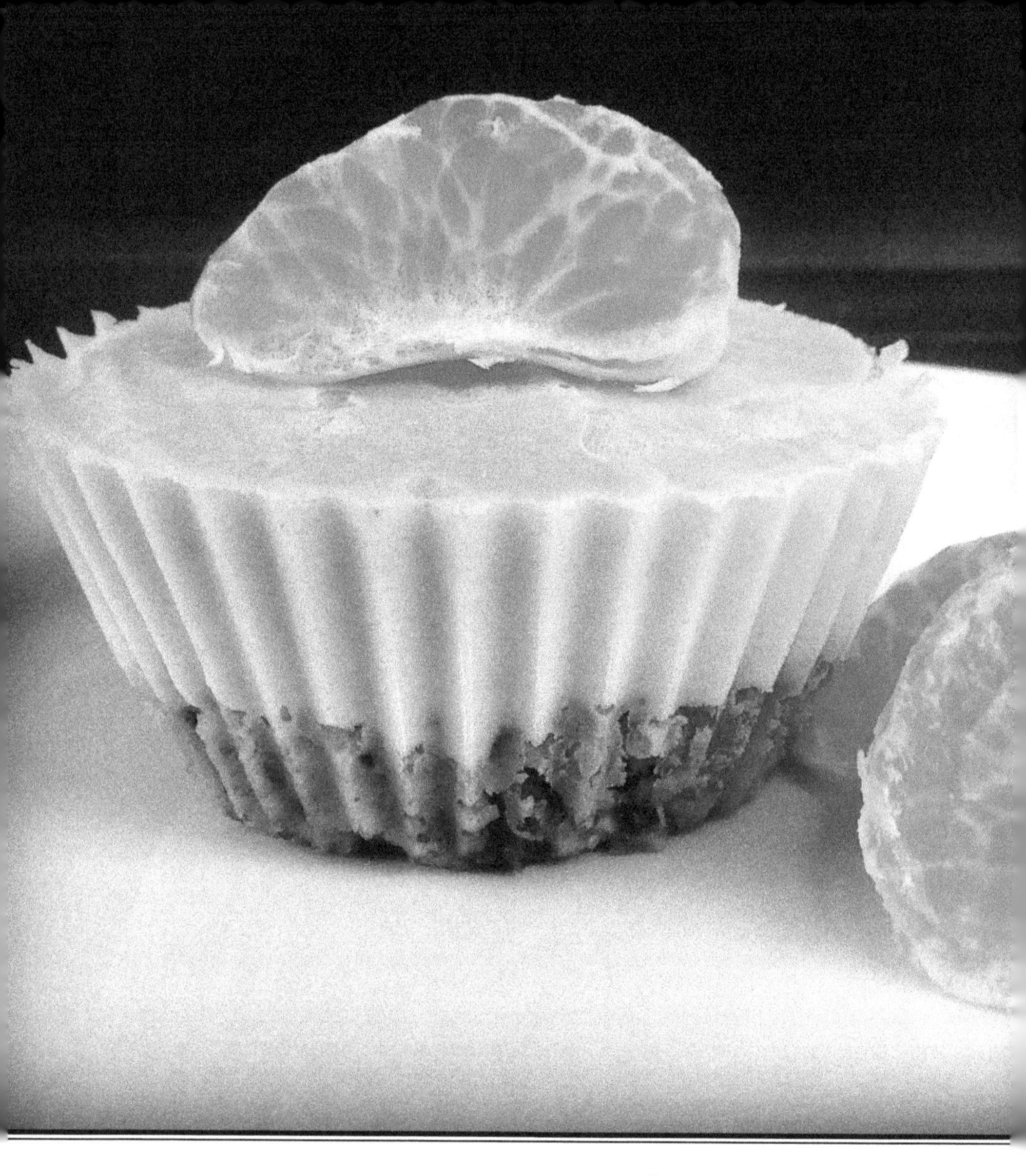

Raw mandarin & orange cheesecake

Come August and September, we always have an abundance of citrus fruit in our garden. I created the recipe for these raw mandarin and orange cheesecakes because our orange trees were simply overflowing with fruit. Raw cakes are great to keep in the freezer, so you can always have a sweet treat on hand.

INGREDIENTS:

Base
1 1/4 cups pecans
1/3 cup medjool dates
2 tablespoons of coconut oil (melted)
2 - 3 drops of vanilla extract
Pinch of Himalayan pink salt

Filling
1 1/2 cup cashews
1 cup mandarin segments (peel removed)
2 cups orange segments (peel removed)
1/4 cup maple syrup
1/3 cup coconut oil (melted then cooled)

METHOD:

Soak cashews for 3-4 hours (see note on previous page).

Process all base ingredients until combined.
Press into 12 silicone moulds in a muffin tray.

Drain cashews and process with mandarin, orange and maple syrup.
Once completely combined, stir through coconut oil.
Share between the 12 silicone moulds (on top of base).
Place in freezer until set.
Store in freezer, however, remove and allow to thaw before eating.

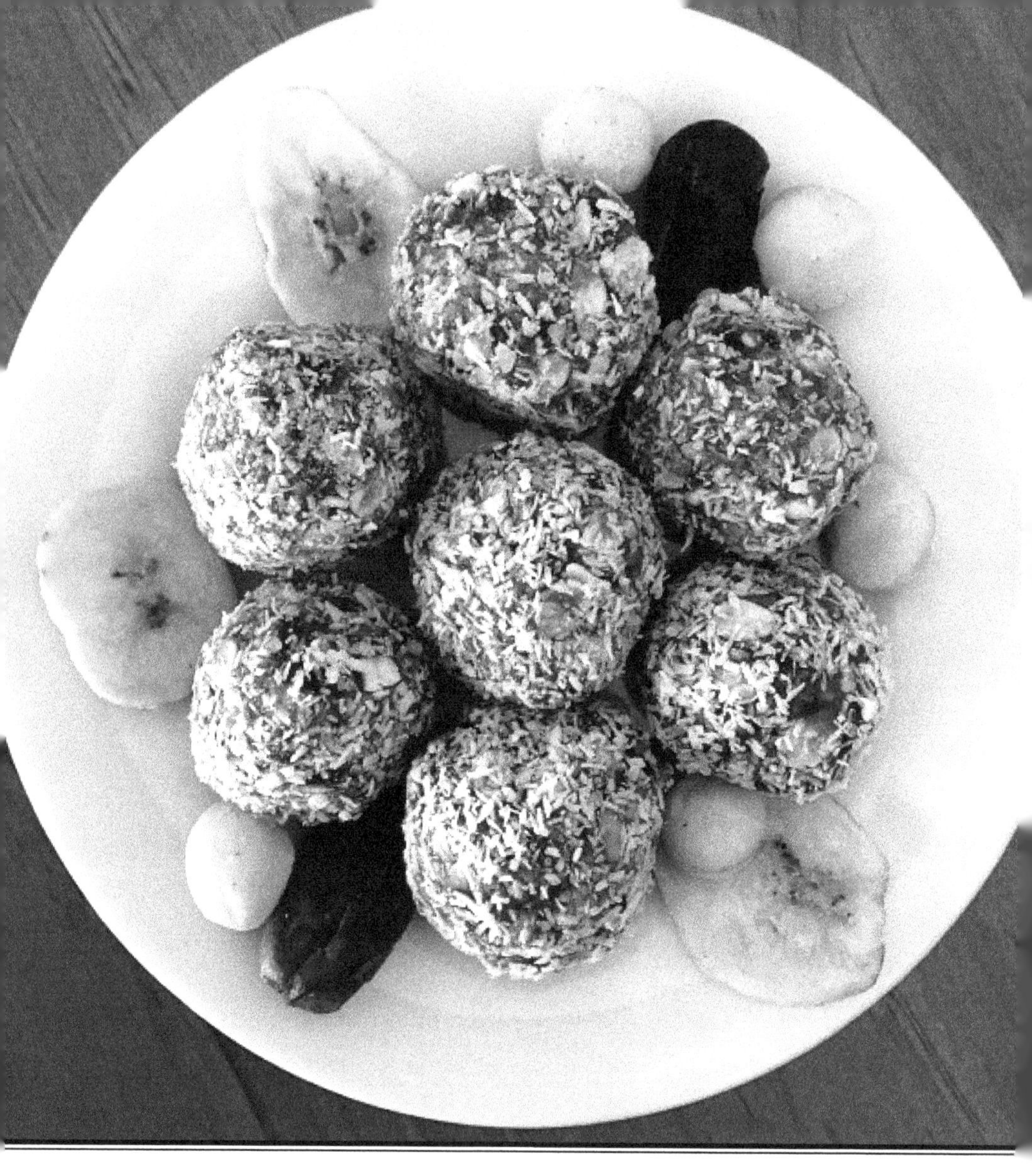

Banoffee bliss balls

Bliss balls are a regular go-to during my weekend prepping sessions. Not only are they quick and easy to make, but you can blitz up so many nutrient-rich ingredients to create handy bite sized snacks. This was one of the first bliss ball recipes I created and they are now a family favourite. Dehydrated banana chips may seem like an unusual ingredient, but combined with dates it creates that beautiful banana-caramel banoffee flavour so many of us enjoy.

INGREDIENTS:

1 cup dehydrated banana chips
10 medjool dates
1/4 cup macadamia nuts
3 tablespoons of cacao
1/4 cup peanut and coconut spread
2 tablespoons melted coconut oil
3/4 cup rolled oats
Desiccated coconut for rolling

METHOD:

Blitz the dehydrated banana chips in the food processor to make a powder. Remove powder and set aside.
Add dates, macadamia nuts, cacao, peanut spread and coconut oil in the food processor (you don't need to wash it after blitzing the banana chips) and process until combined.
In a bowl combine banana powder, processed date mixture and oats, stir until combined.
Roll into balls, then roll in coconut.
Store in the fridge.

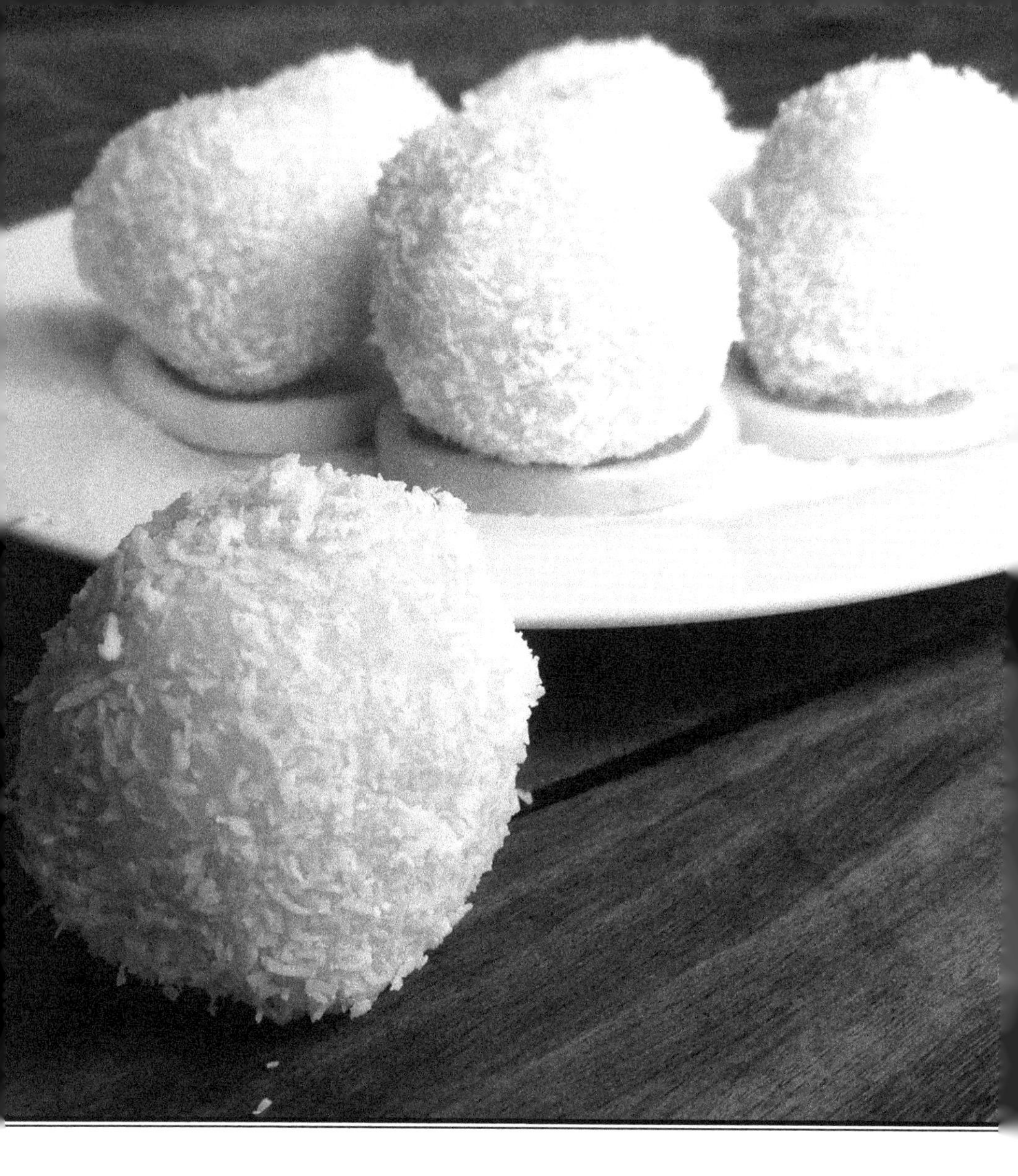

Lemon meringue bliss balls

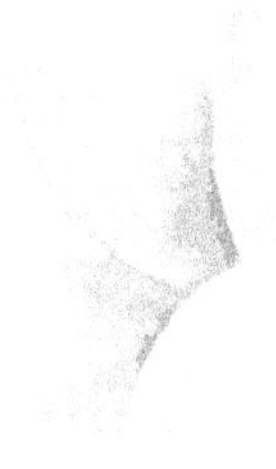

When life gives you lemons, or in this case when your lemon tree gives you oodles of lemons - make Bliss Balls! When citrus fruit is in season, we will always have a bowl full sitting on our side board. Apart from making bliss balls, I love starting the day by adding a slice of lemon to warm water. Or if my boys are feeling a little under the weather, I'll make them a warm lemon, honey and ginger drink. So really, I don't mind too much if life gives me lemons.

INGREDIENTS:

1 cup almond meal
1 1/2 cups desiccated coconut
Juice and rind of 2 lemons
1/3 cup melted coconut oil
1/4 cup agave
1/4 cup additional desiccated coconut

METHOD:

Combine almond meal, coconut, lemon juice and rind, coconut oil and agave in the food processor and blitz until combined.
Shape mixture into balls and roll in additional coconut.
Allow to set in the fridge.

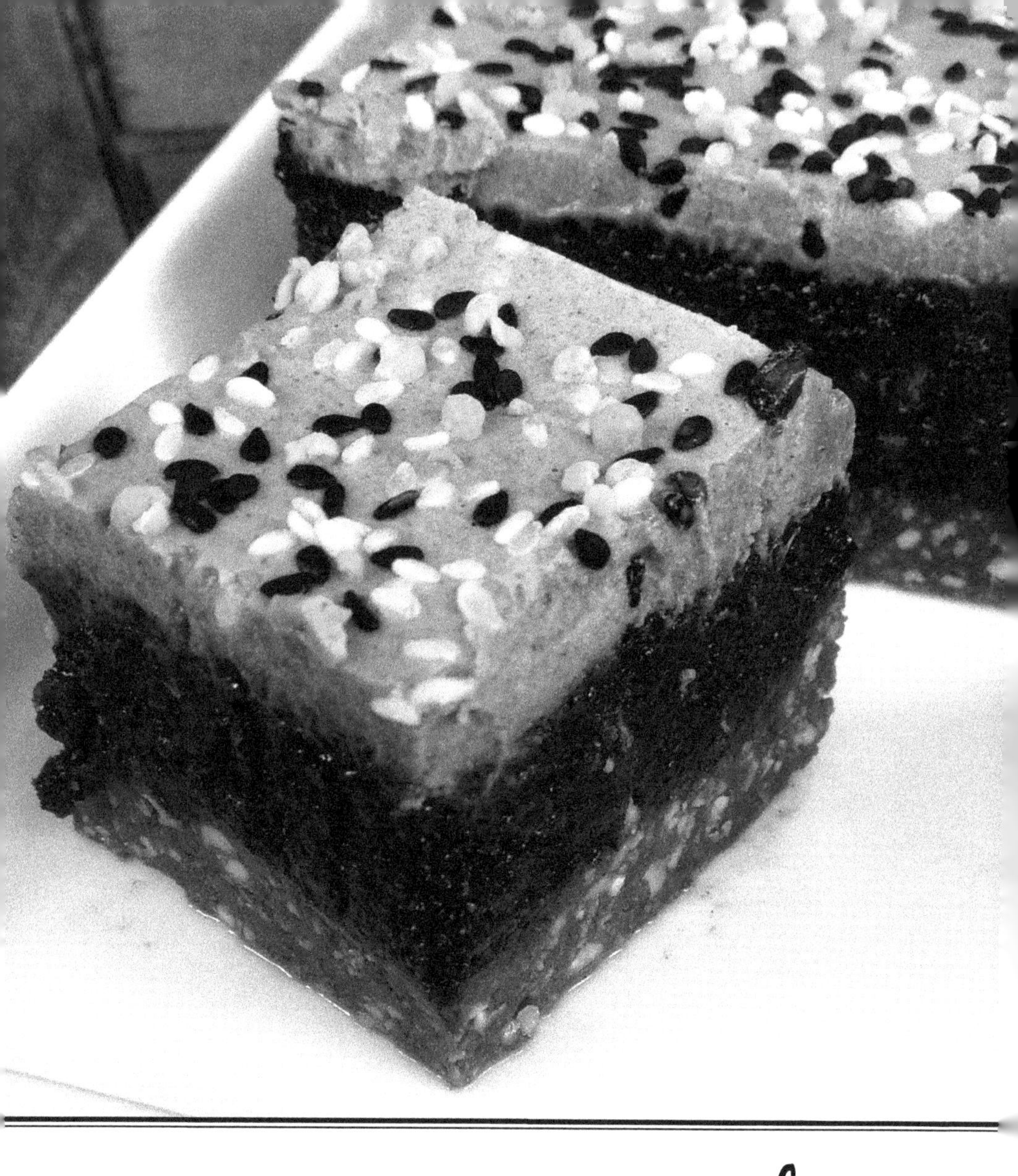

Black tahini slice

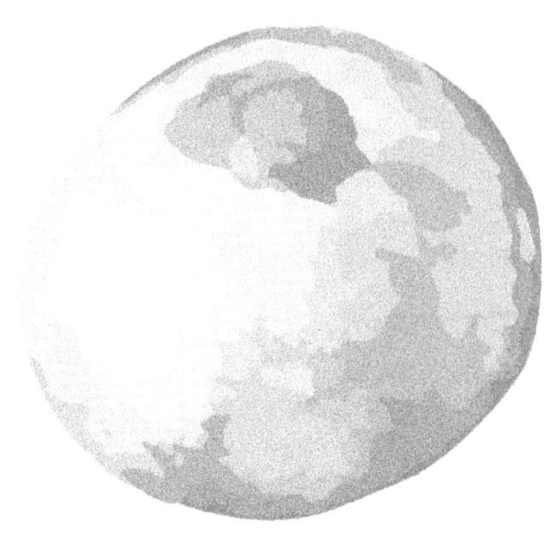

I am a bit of a shop-a-holic when it comes to foodie products. I love health food shops, gourmet food shops and markets - I'll always walk away with something ... even if I'm not quite sure what to do with it. This was the case with my jar of black tahini (a paste made from black sesame seeds). It sat in my pantry for a while, until one day I decided to get inventive. The result was this slice, which is rich and fudgy and will put an end to any chocolate craving you might have!

INGREDIENTS:

Base
1 cup of cashews
1/2 cup pecans
2 tablespoons cacao
1 tablespoon melted coconut oil
1/4 cup coconut syrup

Filling
10 medjool dates
1/2 cup black tahini
2 tablespoon melted coconut oil

Topping
3 tablespoon cacao butter
1/4 cup coconut cream
2 tablespoon coconut syrup
1 tbsp cacao

METHOD:

Base
Process all ingredients until well combined, press into a container. Place into fridge or freezer.

Filling
Process all ingredients until combined. Spread over base. Return to the fridge.

Topping
Melt cacao butter, allow to cool slightly. Stir through cacao, coconut syrup and coconut cream.

Optional: Sprinkle with black and white sesame seeds and bee pollen to decorate.

Matcha slice

This slice ticks all the boxes. It is vegan, gluten, dairy and refined sugar free not to mention packed full of antioxidants AND the filling tastes like a decadent chocolate pudding! The beautiful green colour in the top layer comes from the addition of matcha powder, a finely ground powder made from green tea, which is known as an antioxidant rich food. Store this slice in the freezer, ready to grab as a healthy lunchbox snack.

INGREDIENTS:

Base
1/2 cup cashews
1/2 cup macadamias
2 tablespoons melted coconut oil
1 tablespoon agave
1 teaspoon vanilla paste

Filling
15 medjool dates
2 tablespoons coconut oil
1/3 cup cacao and peanut spread

Top
3 tablespoons cacao butter
3 tablespoons coconut oil
1 teaspoon matcha green tea powder
2 tablespoons agave

METHOD:

Combine base ingredients in the food processor. Press into a tray lined with baking paper and place in the freezer.

Combine filling ingredients in the food processor. Spread over base.
Return to freezer.
(You can use the same food processor, without washing in between to make it a little easier)

Melt cacao butter and coconut oil over low heat until liquid.
Allow to cool for 10 - 15 minutes.
Whisk in coconut cream and matcha.
Pour over slice and allow to set in freezer.

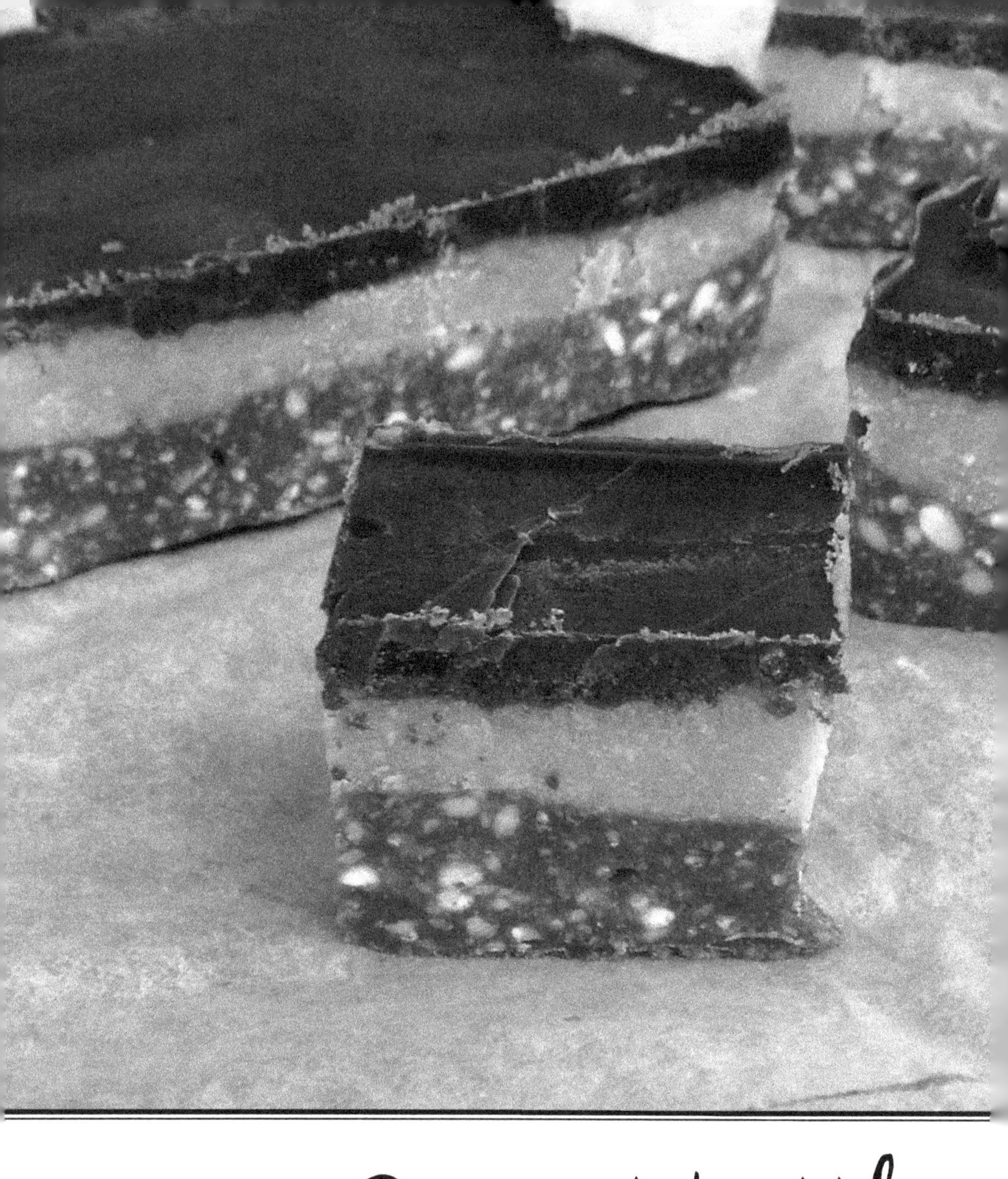

Peanut brittle fudge slice

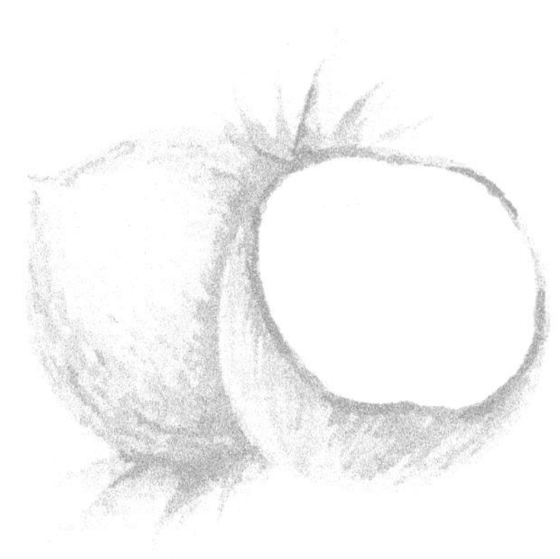

The best thing about this slice, which by the way I didn't plan, is that the coconut syrup in the base somehow sets into toffee like shards. Combined with the peanut butter and the cacao chocolate layer, the flavour combination reminds me of peanut brittle. This version may be made with more wholesome ingredients, but even so, it is quite decadent!

INGREDIENTS:

Base
1 1/2 cup cashews
1/4 cup coconut syrup
1/4 cup cacao
2 tablespoons coconut oil

Filling
1/2 cup all natural peanut butter
1/4 cup coconut syrup
1 tablespoon melted coconut oil

Top
1/4 cup melted coconut oil
1/4 cup cacao
1/4 cup maple syrup

METHOD:

Process all base ingredients until combined.
Press into a square tin, place in freezer.

Process all filling ingredients until combined.
Spread over base and return to freezer.

Whisk top ingredients until combined.
Pour over base and filling.
Return to freezer until set.

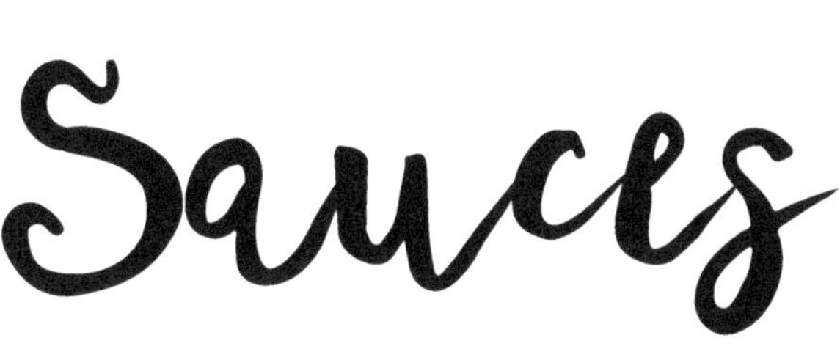

Adding a dressing to your salad means you are adding oodles of flavour. Some people may think a salad for lunch each day is a bore, but with the right dressing, you will be enjoying a tasty and satisfying meal. I tend not to buy pre-made dressings from the supermarket – but I will sometimes indulge in a good quality salad dressing, vinegar or glaze sold at the Farmers' Market or specialty stores - so it is worth keeping an eye out for one that appeals to you.

I pack a small pot of dressing with our salads each day and my quick and easy option is to pack balsamic vinegar. I always have a bottle of both red and white in my pantry. I tend to use the white more regularly as it pairs well with almost any salad. However, I love using the red balsamic when our salads contain tomatoes or feta cheese, the flavours work so well together.

I also love to make my own salad dressing and in this section I will share two of our family favourites. I like to make salad dressings in a screw top jar, which can be kept in the refrigerator to use throughout the week. Just shake before use.

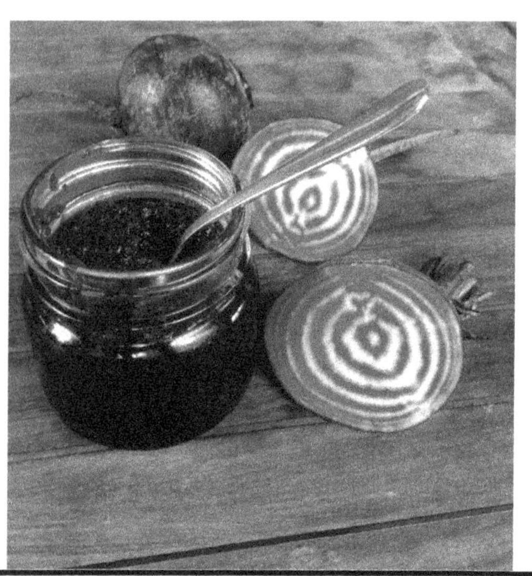

Beetroot relish

Asian dressing

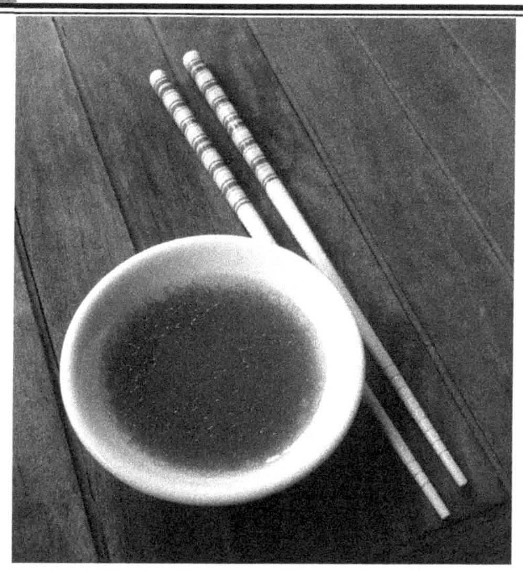

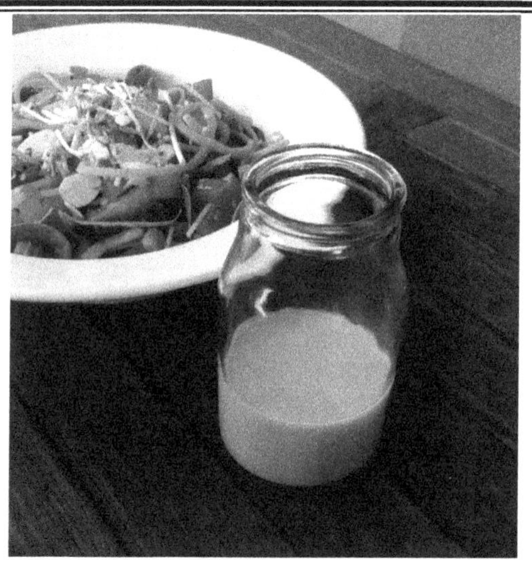

Honey mustard dressing

This recipe was given to me by mum, who got it from my Aunty Jennie - it is delicious!

INGREDIENTS:

750g beetroot
1 brown onion
2 cups sugar
2 cups balsamic vinegar
1 cup water
3 teaspoon yellow mustard seeds
Pinch of brown cloves
5 cm piece orange rind
Sea salt and cracked pepper

METHOD:

Peel and process beetroot and onion.
In a covered fry pan, fry mustard seeds in a little oil.
Add all other ingredients.
Place over medium heat, cover and bring to the boil.
Cook uncovered until beetroot is soft and liquid has reduced and thickened slightly.
Pour into sterilised jars, seal and cool.
Refrigerate after opening.

My entire family love this dressing, probably because it is so sweet. I can literally put this on any salad and they will devour it.

INGREDIENTS:

3 tablespoons lemon juice
1 tablespoon sweet chilli
1 tablespoon soy sauce
1 tablespoon brown sugar
1 tablespoon olive oil

METHOD:

Combine all ingredients in a small jar and shake to combine.
Pour over salad just before serving.

I first made this dressing to go with an apple salad. It was so popular with the boys that I now make it regularly.

INGREDIENTS:

1/3 cup extra-virgin olive oil
1/4 cup white wine vinegar
2 tablespoon Dijon mustard
1 garlic clove (crushed)
1 teaspoon honey

METHOD:

Combine all ingredients in a small jar and shake to combine.
Pour over salad just before serving.

Index

1 + 1 + 1 Slice 29, 36, 41, 45, **100**
Ajvar (Paprika relish) 70
Almonds 30, 35, 48, 55
Apple 32, 37, 68
Apricot 36, 76
Apricot balls 48
Asian Dressing 32, 48, 51, 59, 69, 75, **126**
Banana Bread 33, 64, **98**
Banoffee Bliss Balls 47, 50, 57, **114**
Basics 18
Beetroot chips 43, 44
Beetroot Relish 29, 30,31, 42, 69, 72, 74, 76, **126**
Beetroot Soup 50, 60, **88**
Bek's Date & Nut Slice 30, 37, 51, **100**
Berries:
Blackberries 71
Blueberries 31, 70
Cranberries 50, 76
Goji 59
Strawberries 37, 40, 47, 56, 57, 58, 59, 61, 62, 65, 68, 69, 70, 74, 75, 77
White mulberries 68, 77
Black rice 62
Black rice biscuits 27, 32, 36, 46
Black Tahini Slice 27, 28, 31, 32, **118**
Bliss balls, Banoffee 47, 50, 57, **114**
Lemon meringue 46, 60, 62, **116**
Blueberries 31
Brazil nuts 26, 34, 35, 40, 42, 46, 84
Bread 35, 55, 56
Broccoli 70
Broccoli Nuggets 61, 65, **90**
Brown rice 51, 59
Carrots 26, 30, 33, 35, 36, 41, 46, 47, 49, 51, 54, 65, 69, 70, 71, 72, 73, 77, 79
Carrots, Heirloom 26, 30
Cashews 44, 46, 60, 62, 65, 68
Celery 58
Cheese:
Chedder 30, 46, 74
Feta 40
Goats 55, 57
Haloumi 31
Cherries 61, 64
Cherry tomatoes 27
Chocolate Crackles 43, 72, 75, 78, **108**
Choc-rice Slice 40, **106**
Coconut chips 55
Corn chips 40, 47, 78
Couscous 79
Crackers 30, 41, 61, 62, 74
Crisps 45, 48, 60
Cucumber 46, 74
Dark chocolate 64
Dip 26, 35, 36, 49, 51, 56, 60, 61, 62, 71, 73, 75, 77
Dressing:
Asian 32, 48, 51, 59, 69, 75, **126**
Honey mustard 34, 43, 45, 74, **126**
Edamame beans 59
Eggplant 36
Fig, Raw Cheesecake 44, 55, 57, **110**
Fruit Leather 27, 32, 34, 35, 48, **96**
Fruit loaf 34, **96**
Funfetti protein slice 34, 35, **104**
Grapes 26, 30, 31, 42, 48, 49
Grapes, Crimson 45, 46, 54, 59
Gyoza 75
Healthy packet mix snacks 69, 77
Heirloom carrots, 26, 30
Herby Chickpea Crackers 69, 70, **92**

Honey mustard dressing 34, 43, 45, 74, **126**
Hummus 41, 47, 77
Jackfruit, Pulled 47, 48, **86**
Kiwi Fruit 28, 43, 44, 55, 60, 62, 63, 64, 65, 70, 73, 75, 78, 79
Kri Kri 28, 76
Lemon Meringue Bliss Balls 46, 60, 62, **116**
Lentils 34, 37, 56, 60, 61
Lunchbox Tips 22
Macadamia nuts 32, 47, 64, 78
Mandarin 45, 57, 58
Mandarin, Raw Cheesecake 68, 74, 79, **112**
Matcha Choc-Fudge Slice 48, 49, 56, 58, 70, **120**
Meal Planner 14
Mizuna 43, 49, 71
Nectarine 32, 74
Nougat 78
Nut Loaf 44, 62, **84**
Nuts:
- Almonds 30, 35, 48, 55
- Brazil Nuts 26, 34, 35, 40, 42, 46, 84
- Cashews 44, 46, 60, 62, 65, 68
- Macadamia 32, 47, 64, 78
- Peanuts 49
- Pistachios 27, 29, 31, 57

Orange 68
Orange, Raw Cheesecake **112**
Passionfruit 28, 40, 41, 46
Peach 27
Peanuts 49
Peanut Brittle Fudge Slice **122**
Pear 55
Pineapple 34, 51, 70, 71, 72
Pistachio nuts 27, 29, 31, 57
Plums 29, 33, 34, 35, 41, 47, 69
Pomegranate 36
Popcorn 32, 71
Pumpkin seed oil 49
Pumpkin seeds 32, 50, 56, 61, 65, 74
Preparation 14
Pulled Jackfruit **86**
Quinoa 64, 65
Quinoa sticks 64
Raw Fig Cheescake 44, 55, 57, **110**
Raw Mandarin & Orange Cheesecake 68, 74, 79, **112**
Rice, Black 62
Rice, Brown 51, 59
Rice, Wild 48
Salad:
- Bean/lentil 34, 37, 56, 60, 61
- Cheese 30, 31, 40, 55, 57, 78, 79
- Noodle 47, 69
- Pasta 27, 42, 49, 64, 79
- Rice 48, 51, 59, 62, 64, 74
- Roast vegetable 28, 29, 30, 33, 36, 37, 50, 72
- Steamed vegetable 56, 70
- Tofu 32

Saukraut 58
Snow peas 44, 76
Storage 20
Sultanas 31
Sunflower seeds 71
Sweet potato 57
Sweet potato sushi 57, 63
Sushi, sweet potato 57, 63
Tofu 32
Tomatoes 37
Tomatoes, Cherry 27
Trail mix 33, 41, 51, 54, 72, 79
Vegetable crisps 37, 45, 56, 73, 75
Vegetable chips 26, 50, 58, 62
Vegetable straws 29, 31
Veggie 'Sausage' Rolls 28, **82**
Watermelon 42, 77
Wild rice 48
Wraps 43, 49
Zoodles 28, 41
Zucchini 28, 35, 41

Acknowledgements

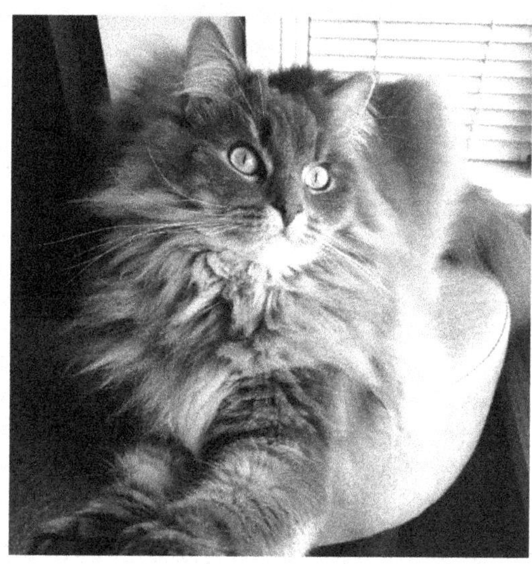

It has been quite a journey from my first foodie photos (taken covertly, hoping no one would see) to holding this book in my hands. The support I have received from all of my family and friends has been amazing and there a few people I'd specifically like to thank.

My parents who have been a constant source of encouragement and support. And, who still have me around for dinner every week.

My friends, who listened to me, offered me advice, and who have gone on foodie adventures with me. Meditation retreats, vegan festivals, road trips to try cafés or on health food and market tours – you know who you are!

The amazing people I have discovered through Instagram. It has been wonderful to connect with so many like-minded souls from all around the globe. I am constantly inspired and motivated by this ever growing community and those who follow my account.

Finally, thank you to my husband Brendan, and my children Caiden and Logan. Thank you for trying all of my creations and for always giving me your (very) honest feedback. Thank you for humouring me while I show you countless pictures of food or lunch box arrangements seeking your opinion. But most of all, thank you for believing in me and supporting me on this journey.

About Renae

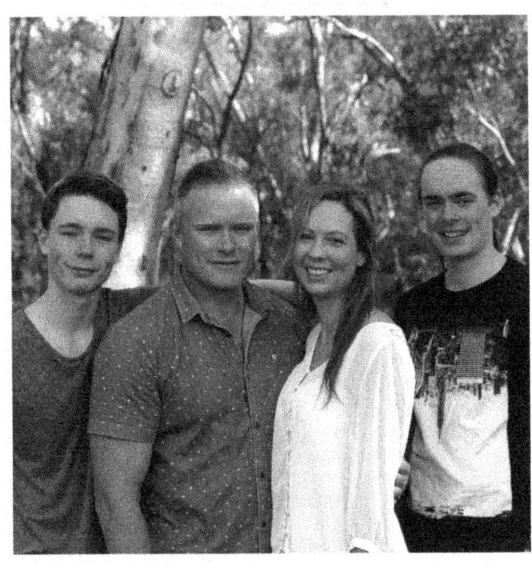

Renae Westley is a primary school teacher, wife and mother of two boys. She has been a vegetarian for almost 10 years. After searching for vegetarian inspiration on Instagram, she was decided to get involved and create one of her own in order to share her food journey (and so as not to bore her friends who may have been following her personal account!) In 2013, @lifeofavegetarian was born.

By then end of 2014, the account had over 10,000 followers and one year later it had over 35,000. With well over 50,000 followers by mid-2016, Renae realised that many other people, from all over the globe, were keen to be inspired and to get creative with their vegetarian lunches!

Renae says that she thinks lunchtime is often the forgotten meal - the one that is rushed or thought of (and consumed) at the last minute. Her lunchboxes prove that a vegetarian lunch doesn't have to be boring and it is a joy to send your loved ones off for the day with a healthy, nutritious and beautiful meal.

CPSIA information can be obtained
at www.ICGtesting.com
Printed in the USA
BVHW06s1716010618
517845BV00014B/95/P

9 780994 412621